TALKING ABOUT
HOMOEOPATHY

TALKING ABOUT HOMOEOPATHY

Dr. Trevor Smith

M.A., M.B. Chir., D.P.M., M.F. Hom.

Insight Editions
WORTHING, Sussex
1986

First published 1986

© Trevor Smith 1986

British Library Cataloguing in Publication Data

Smith, Trevor, *1934*-
    Talking about homeopathy.
    1. Homeopathy
    I. Title
    615.5'32   RX71

WARNING
The contents of this volume are for general interest only and individual persons should always consult their medical adviser about a particular problem or before stopping or changing an existing treatment.

ISBN 0 946670 10 2

Typeset by Acorn Bookwork, Salisbury, Wiltshire
Printed and bound in Great Britain by
Biddles, Guildford, Surrey

Contents

Preface

I have aimed in Talking about Homoeopathy, to bring together a contrasting and varied series of talks and articles given over the past five years. Several have already appeared in Homoeopathy and Homoeopathy Today, and others have not been previously published or heard. The aim has been to produce a volume of overall interest and viewpoint, in a wide variety of areas, which would be impossible in any single lecture, article or talk and to stimulate a maximum of thought and discussion. The results of a double-blind proving experiment with Kali Carb. are included, also a series of varied articles on the psychological aspects of homoeopathy in various emotional conditions – a little known role for the method, which I consider of major importance to every practitioner. Included also are a series of talks given to the Winchester Homoeopathic Society for the newcomer to Homoeopathy, with notes on the twenty basic potencies for the family medicine chest including holiday and first-aid remedies.

In the chapter on the causation of illness, I have given my view on the deeper, more subtle factors, which play a causative role in disease. Other more theoretical articles are concerned with the generalized application of the similimum principles, homoeopathic potencies and on the difficulties of self-prescribing. A series of articles deals with the most common emotional problems which many families will have experienced in at least one member at some time. The major remedies for insomnia, grief, and tension are of general interest, for both patient and practitioner. The chapters on homoeopathic nosodes and schizophrenia are more specialised, but hopefully also of some general interest.

In all the discussions, I have tried to bring together my personal views, based on clinical experience working with patients and the importance of the mentals, for everyday practice and dealing with the ordinary problems which arise in the surgery.

I have always found the psychologicals to be of importance, for both physical as well as the more obvious emotional problems, not only because of my particular interest and background in psychiatry, but essentially from clinical experience and day to day working with the individuals of every age and often families. A detailed history, including the origins and salient psychological features of trigger-factors is invaluable, both as an aid to more accurate prescribing and to potency levels.

When all other previous treatments have failed, the right homoeopathic remedy in the correct potency is often curative, but awareness of depth of each problem and any emotional associations, gives an added insight and depth to both communication and understanding and the key doctor–patient relationship.

1

Talking about Homoeopathy

Homoeopathy is a method of treatment, over 200 years old which took origin in Germany through the insights of a rather unusual physician who was based in Meissen. His name was Samuel Hahnemann, and he developed some very old principles, which although known since Hippocrates, had not been clinically used until he rediscovered them – much as Freud did with the unconscious. The genius of Hahnemann, the Father of Homoeopathy was to test-out in the consulting room, a totally new way of looking at people and their illness.

The homoeopath differs from his colleagues in the way he prescribes, but also in the way he or she looks at a patient. In homoeopathy we take a holistic viewpoint and look at the whole patient and person – often the whole family over several generations. The remedies used are natural, mostly of plant origin, but some are also from mineral and animal sources. Homoeopathy does not use anything inert or synthetic, unless there is a specific indication to do so. Most of the remedies are toxic

1

when undiluted, and can stimulate a massive physiological reaction. For example, Deadly Nightshade, taken from the hedgerow evokes a very powerful, and usually unpleasant overall body reaction. But in its homoeopathic form of *Belladonna*, the reaction, although generalized, is controlled and directed, to evoke a healing response in a particular and specific area of the body. Homoeopathy works on simple principles, which are inherent in its name. The Greek word homoeopathy means similar or equal pathos or suffering. The principle of 'Let like be treated by like' is often expressed by the Latin phrase – *similia, similibus curentur*, which succinctly describe the method. The homoeopath is a specialist in comparing the toxic picture of the remedies with the symptoms of the patient and using the comparison to predict and prescribe a remedy-reaction best suited to the individual patient.

A child seen today, had feverish pain in the right ear, the skin hot and sweating, and generally over-active and anxious. I examined the ear which was tender and painful and saw a red, tense, inflamed ear drum, the blood vessels dilated and obviously in an active state. The diagnosis was otitis media or acute middle-ear infection. *Belladonna* was prescribed, because *Belladonna* poisoning matched the characteristics of the case. There was a fast pulse, a hot, red face, general agitation, and dilated pupils from anxiety, apprehension and pain. In other cases it is often the throat which is affected where *Belladonna* is most indicated.

You may ask – how does homoeopathy differ from allopathic or conventional medicine, where an opposite medicine is prescribed – a pain killer for headache, an anti-spasmodic for pain, or an anti-depressant for a depression. In homoeopathy we only match the symptoms of the patient to those of a remedy under consideration, the pre-scriber does not suppress symptoms, because he or she believes that it is a short-term approach, and ultimately harmful to the patient.

The reasons why the child developed an ear infection are interesting too. The mother said, 'She is at playschool, having lunches once a week, and she has become terrified because she has to finish them, or she will be told off by the headmistress who's a bit of a dragon – the child is terrified.' She asked me 'Should I force her to have lunches or not?' I replied 'No – go and talk to the headmis-tress, but don't force her.' Once the child is five, she has to take school lunches, but until that age they are voluntary. In this instance, anxiety, even terror, was undermining the child's resistance and she was getting recurrent earache.

Hahnemann emphasized the fundamental importance and the key role of stress in illness. I am not implying that all illness is stress-produced, because it is not. But stress is always a very power-ful factor in illnesses at every age. The child didn't come with a psychological condition – she was crying because of a very painful earache, but she was also crying with fear inside herself. Here an ordinary, common, physical condition, when given time, showed the underlying causes, which could then be talked about and resolved. The emergence of depth perspectives, and understanding, the reasons behind a problem is also one of the major concerns of the homoeopathic method.

Stress depletes vital reserves and makes for ill-ness at any age. At the age of four, when vital defensive energy is depleted, you may get earache. At the age of eleven it may be a sore throat. By fifteen – acne may be more common and by twenty there may be asthma or sinus catarrh. The adult of thirty-five may show his or her depleted resistance by recurrent winter bronchitis. We are all susceptible to stress at different ages and levels of maturity reacting in different ways at each stage. At forty stress may induce pre-menstrual tension, or a peptic ulcer.

Hahnemann was a rebel, and did not go along with the conventional approach of purgation and blood-letting treatments of his time. He thought they were depleting to the patient, and more damaging than curative. When translating a major work by the Scottish physician Cullen, concerning the treatment of malaria, he became dissatisfied with the treatments described. He decided to experiment and took quinine himself, using natural Cinchona bark tincture, from which it is extracted. In a short time he developed all the symptoms of a malaria-like illness – intermittent fever, weakness and rigors. This made him think that if Cinchona can cause the malarial-like symptoms, it can also cure them. As soon as Hahnemann stopped taking the Cinchona, the symptoms disappeared and he was perfectly well.

In this way and from these origins, Hahnemann developed about 200 remedies with the help of a small group of followers. He found that if he gave the undiluted mother tincture of the remedy, like a strong herbal remedy, patients developed side-effects. He began to dilute the remedies and found paradoxically that this increased their efficacy, their power or potency instead of the opposite. The more he diluted, the stronger the therapeutic effect obtained. This is unique to homoeopathy, not only about the way of thinking about the patient – but also the preparation of the remedies. The diluted remedy is safe, there is no risk in homoeopathy and a patient is not harmed by his or her treatment. One drop of mother tincture in 99 drops of dilutant fluid gives the first centesimal dilution, and when repeated six times, this gives the 6th centesimal or 6c strength, a dilution of 10^{-12}. The 6c potency is one which is commonly used for the first-aid and local problems and one which is valuable for home use.

No one knows exactly how homoeopathy works, but it is based on energy release, the freeing of vitality blocks at cellular and tissue levels. Man does not naturally respond to substances en masse, but is more biologically attuned to a small stimulus which is in harmony with the body's needs. When prescribing homoeopathic remedies in high potency, it is no longer the substance which is effective, but the energy of the remedy in solution. At present, this may seem inexplicable, but there are many scientific fields where the minute, and the unmeasurable, has an effect, often overwhelmingly so, particularly in the field of toxicology, chemical and pesticide leakage and atmospheric pollution. Arsenic fed to yeast cell cultures in a medium dose only inhibits growth, a massive dose kills the cells, but the minutest amount is a stimulus to growth.

When there is a surgical condition, homoeo-pathy is not usually indicated. But it will help prepare the patient for the operation (*Arnica*) and smooth the recovery period (*Staphysagia*). The homoeopath thinks of the patient first, not of any homoeopathic principles and homoeopathy has never been a cure-for-all-illness or a panacea. Like any aspect of medicine, it should not be idealized or an end in itself. Homoeopathy often resolves emotional or mental problems as well as the physical, provided enough time is given to the patient and there is careful prescribing of the correct potency and the right remedy.

In childbirth, unless there is an obstructive problem – a narrow or flat pelvis, requiring surgical relief or instrument assistance, or where the head does not engage, homoeopathy can also help to stimulate healthy uterine tone and an uncomplicated delivery (*Caulophyllum*). *Arnica* also helps in childbirth for problems of shock, loss of blood and psychological distress.

Homoeopathy usually takes time because the remedies work on the subtle energy levels of the patient. Hahnemann called it vital energy but others prefer the term defensive energy.

A man of 56 came with severe varicose veins. The veins were black, irregular and pouching, the size of small pigeon eggs. There was considerable aching along the veins, especially after walking. I prescribed *Hammamelis* (Witch Hazel). A fortnight later a friend of the family telephoned to say 'What have you done to Mr. A. – he's in a terrible state, his legs are painful and cannot walk'. When I saw the patient however, the whole of the affected vein had firmed and tightened. There was hardly any pouching visible, and the whole varicose condition had almost resolved. The 'pain' complained of, was the increase of healthy tone in the vein, and not due to any worsening of the condition or a new problem developing. I normally allow six months for a varicose condition to improve, but this man had achieved it in four weeks.

With some patients, resolution of a problem

happens quickly, but the speed and response of reaction is always a very individual thing. The length of time a treatment takes to cure is often unknown, because of the many depths and levels to every disorder and the associated personality of the person involved. The homoeopathic remedy can and does encompass all these levels of the patient and this is why the results are so effective, often seeming even to be dramatic.

2

On the Nature of Illness

The deeper, subtle aspects of homoeopathy are not easily defined. They are less describable than the consistency of sputum, characteristics of a cough or colour of a rash which give a pointer to diagnosis. The deeper aspects of illness, with which homoeopathy is concerned, are the more personal, often psychological ones, and when talking about the emotional aspects, you also have to acknowledge the spiritual too, because they are inseparable.

The word I prefer for spiritual is existential, because it is closer to what the person actually experiences of it. When thinking about the psychologicals and the deeper factors in illness, the question one wants to ask is not just – 'what are the manifestations of a cold – but why did it happen?' There are many unknowns as to why someone catches a cold on a particular day and also many questions as to why a person gets ill in a particular way. Often we do not know the answer or can only hazard a guess. It is usually just accepted that someone gets ill in a particular week or on a certain day. But some are ill at a particular time every year, always ill in the Spring or Summer – an anniversary reaction perhaps, but often from no obvious psychological reason. When this happens, a family may often say 'Jim is a bit accident-prone', or 'Aunty gets her annual attack of rheumatism or gout every Spring – it's her nature, body clock or perhaps her karma'. On other occasions the clues are clearer, and the exact trigger factor causing the illness is clearer. Since Janet's engagement was broken, her hair has gone grey in six weeks, or Bill has developed a smoker's cough since he was made redundant, or Anne's periods have become painful since her mother died. Ever since Wynn lost her sister from cancer, she has become more depressed and more irritable. What makes for susceptibility to illness, accident-proneness, vulnerability and a lowering of resistance often seems to be an acute psychological trauma of some kind – but does it only exist in the mind as a fixed idea or is it a form of changed resistance to life and growth? Is there even a reality to any depth of illness existing? – other than the superficial rash, the running nose, or a burning throat? Another interesting question is – 'Can a synthetic remedy, without life or vitality, *really* reach, resonate and harmonize with a sickness process within the person and in any depth?

Some will say there is no such thing as sickness other than in the body and that any changes of imagination and feelings are purely secondary effects. But allergic conditions associated quite scientifically with a foreign protein reaction can also be inhibited or cancelled by hypnosis. The Mantoux, tuberculous-sensitivity reaction is one of the deepest allergic reactions known, testing previous infection, but it can be stopped by suggestion under the hypnotic trance.

We know beyond reasonable doubt that every

9

person unquestionably has various depths and layers to their level of thinking, feelings and reaction, but are these relevant to illness? Do they play a role at all? Such layers are usually quite clearly seen and known about. When people turn away from a conventional way of thinking, away from fixed dogma, absolute faith or certainties in any area, they nevertheless usually embrace something else, rather similar, with just as much fervour and dogmatism as before. A person who has turned against the dictates of the church usually embraces the dogma of another organization with equal certainty and unquestionable knowing. The need to express such needs and controls without question has just taken another form. When a teenager rebels against adult clothes and life-style, they often become equally uniform and conventional in their own dress and hairstyle.

Homoeopathic remedies are alive, not synthetic and 'dead' adynamic mixtures. In the higher potencies, although there is no measurable molecule of original substance left, their pattern of intrinsic energy remains and can evoke a powerful, healing reaction. It is this intrinsic energy which gives uniqueness to each remedy and allows it to reach the deeper psychological aspects. In every illness without exception there is also a psychological factor present, whatever the age or form of disease.

When a patient is given a remedy in a high enough potency, the causative factors often emerge, sometimes over a period of weeks or longer as the remedy frees any psychological hang-ups which have been fixed in depth within the personality.

A man in his seventies with a prostatic problem

came for treatment. It is easy to think that the cause was his age. But he said that what had caused the recent symptoms was being obliged to make redundant a lot of loyal men who had been with him for twenty years or more. Deep feelings of regret and guilt profoundly upset him and set off his prostate. It was not really that he had a prostate problem but one of anguish and the urinary symptoms were only the most superficial features of the true cause.

Another patient came recently because of an allergy to a well-known foam bath preparation. She had used the same one for many years, and it did not make sense that she should have a problem with it now. There was a severe urticarial reaction however, aggravated by any detergents she used. The allergy did not make sense, neither to her nor to her family. Only when she was leaving did she talk about her daughter-in-law, her pregnancy and that she had nearly died in hospital, almost lost the baby, with enormous stress at that time. Only the link of stress and the foam bath made sense of the severe and disturbed over-reaction within her skin at that time.

Such factors are usually known about within a sensitive, more open family. Mothers know about it with their children. Often more than one factor is present and these link up to form a stimulus or illness. Within the spiritual aspects of the individual, it is often impossible to formulate questions or answers, and if you do try to do so, it is easy to get it wrong. Most people formulate something which reflects them or which takes them away from a problem, rather than any deeper meaning. Sometimes you have to accept that there are some things you cannot put into words easily, or even talk about – especially very deep personal layers of being and feeling. Part of the problem in talking about the emotional, is that at the same time we also are talking about the inspirational and the indefinable. Loss of faith, or alienation from the spiritual is one of the worst experiences that can exist for any one. Loss may be in relation to formal religion or it may be loss of belief in life or conviction about a relationship. When faith goes you may feel yourself totally bereft, because it is a psychological as well as a spiritual loss at the time. Loss of faith causes despair and depression, particularly in the elderly when alone or isolated from friends, family and mobility. To some extent everyone is prone to some anxiety of this kind – about identity, about existing, and being. For many, this awareness is true spirituality, the ability to tolerate existence and some degree of alienation. But when severe, alienation can also turn into depression although not necessarily a psychological depression. Depression is usually concerned with problems of guilt. Alienation problems are different and cause a healthier, although equally painful depression of awareness. Spiritual alienation can make existing emotional problems more severe and anti-depressants, sedatives or tranquillizers may aggravate the problem because they miss the point. The individual may develop a mixed picture of emotional depression and a deeper, suppressed spiritual problem which when recognized and admitted, can lead to a more positive attitude. It is such complex problems as these, that homoeopathy can relieve and put back into a more balanced perspective.

There are no homoeopathic remedies for loss of faith or spiritual alienation, as the prescription

12

depends on the totality of individual reactions and any feelings rather than on any recipe approach to isolated aspects. Homoeopathy brings problem areas to the surface, to a level where they are more available for resolution and cure. Much of homoeopathy is concerned with this process, increasing awareness and availability of symptoms so that the patient can see more clearly the problem, and work out a more individual solution for themselves.

A patient with a schizophrenic problem, no longer acute and now more the victim of having been institutionalized for long periods said 'I have lost my soul, killed off all meaning to life, destroyed my spirituality. This is why I'm ill. God help me!' Here was an example of the acute pain of existential awareness, after a self-destructive, alienating psychotic experience. The ideas seemed depressive, but in fact reflected a much more healthy awareness than the previous delusional state.

A woman in a supermarket came heavily-laden to the check-out point. A cucumber she had chosen, fell from her basket onto the floor and split. She picked it up and took it back to where she had taken it and chose another. She felt at the time that it was wrong but replaced it nevertheless. Later she said that she should have paid for the cucumber and did not know why she didn't, as it only cost thirty pence. At the check-out point she felt terrible. In the street she felt worse, that she had let herself down. An hour later she returned to take it out and pay for it – but it had disappeared. The story describes the levels of her intolerance and her self-perfection. She could not accept the split cucumber, the fact that she had dropped it on the floor and then put it back. The check-out point

13

symbolized consciousness, admission and awareness. She had made a slip only, been a little clumsy,
and we all do this, as we hurt people we care about.
Having made the slip, she did not admit it at the
time and instead of accepting her human error and
paying for it, she denied it and with it herself. She
suppressed, by putting back the cucumber, and
went through without reference to it, feeling awful.
An hour later it was too late to repair the damage –
both to the cucumber and to herself.

The cucumber story is a good example of what
many of us do with inconvenient feelings and
guilts. As soon as something comes up which
doesn't feel quite right or easy, it is put back under
the pile. You may do that in life but you cannot
keep doing it psychologically without developing
some reaction or problem as a result. We all need
to acknowledge being clumsy, imperfect and to feel
guilt, so that it can be repaired. If not, there is
damage which can accumulate and cause illness. In
fact she had done just this many times, and in an
accumulative way it had eventually broken through
as a persistent illness.

Does it matter if you put the cucumber back on
the pile and accept some inadequacy and personal
guilt? It does if such episodes are closely interwo-
ven with the depths of your personality. It matters
if you are undermining yourself or depriving yourself by doing it.

Another patient was in a department store and
was trying to agree some fittings for a bedroom
unit with his wife. She liked one model and he
liked another. The argument was whether the
model chosen would protrude half an inch and
spoil the general effect or not. Nevertheless he

14

agreed and said 'we'll have the one you like' – but he didn't really feel happy about it or genuine. He really liked what he had chosen and instead of saying so, or buying one of each to try at home, he also put it back on the pile and when they were having dinner that evening was very sulky and silent. Had he been more himself, more true to his real feelings and convictions, there would not have been a backlash of negative feelings and irritability later.

Everything needs repairing and being brought to check-out for this sort of acknowledgement and repair. But you cannot repair, if you push it back under the pile because it builds up guilt, and in its wake illness.

Symptoms are the tip of the iceberg. Not infrequently they occur when it is too late for early warning signs to be treated and cured. There may be weeks or months of internal change before an illness manifests, often at a physical level when the problem is repetitive. Every shock or stress undermines vitality to some degree and allows 'dis-ease' to gain a hold or to break through normal defences. Unless these areas of spiritual and psychological vulnerability are dealt with as they occur, they can create an internal split in confidence and identity, so that disease processes take root.

Psychological health accepts the inevitable imperfections of each of us, the slips, errors, vicissitudes, ambivalence, envy, jealousy, competitiveness present as well as the tenderness, concern, loyalty and love.

The homoeopathic remedy can help make such feelings more available and acceptable, turning

self-destructive anxiety or guilt into more meaningful feelings so that they can be integrated and
worked positively into the totality of the individual.

3

The Similimum Principles

The homoeopath considers a psychological disorder to be that condition of the individual where mental symptoms are most predominant within the total symptom picture of that person.

I would like to discuss, briefly, various types of conventional non-homoeopathic treatments which have proved to be of some value in helping psychological disorders over the years, and to suggest the possibility that there is a 'similimum principle' at work, in spite of the approach being far from Hahnemannian in concept, and remedies used. In some of the classical treatments to be mentioned the patient may be considered as a totality, and accepted in a holistic way, but frequently this is not the case, and the predominant aim is relief of symptoms, either with or without suppression of underlying causes.

Non-Homoeopathic Treatments

Abreaction is the first technique I would like to consider. This is a form of treatment which is still used in psychiatry, having been popular since the turn of the century. It is frequently called the 'truth drug' and is a powerful suggestive form of therapy. Freud called it 'catharsis', referring to the often violent emergence of pent-up emotion and excess energy. The outward manifestations may be hysterical and dramatic, though this may be less extreme.

The usual form the treatment takes is to inject a small dosage of a quick acting anaesthetic to create a pre-conscious state of mind and relaxation, with the anaesthesia, and to favour a disassociated state of thinking. Other methods are the injection of sterile water or the inhalation of one of the milder dental anaesthetics, such as nitrous oxide.

In all these techniques, when they are effective, they seem to facilitate the patient to re-create in his mind – the similimum experience – and then to exteriorize it in the outward manifestations of the abreaction. The drug, gas or injection is a 'trigger' mechanism which allows the patient to re-create and re-live in his mind the original traumatic happening. I am calling this the 'similimum experience' – as once this has emerged, there is usually a relief of tension and symptoms, and improvement can then occur, as a result of consciously re-experiencing the original event and associated memories and feelings.

In shell-shocked troops this was very effective, particularly when the traumatic situation was fairly recent, clear-cut and well-defined, and they were people of hitherto healthy personality. These men would re-create all the traumas and fears of the trench and wartime experience, and it was of great value in rehabilitating soldiers, once the blocked emotional experience had come to the surface and been discharged. In the catharsis of the experience, the patient's own vital resources were able to effect a cure – hitherto impossible because of the strength of the repression and blockage.

Child Analysis

Not only in child analysis, but also in healthy child play, can one see children re-creating externally, in order to master, those fears which might otherwise overwhelm and crush their development. The psychotic child is frequently quite unable to play, and therefore overcome anxieties and fears. The play itself has lost its function and becomes a thing to be feared in itself.

I want to suggest that when the little girl throws a doll repeatedly onto the ground from her pram or high chair – she is not only wanting it to be picked up, and seeking attention and reassurance. She is also mastering fears that she will be abandoned and rejected, perhaps because of her ambivalence to a new baby, or her rage about weaning. By throwing the doll, she is also creating a 'similimum experience' to allow her to grow and develop. She needs to throw that doll on the ground repeatedly, whenever it is handed back to her, and she may need to break it. She thereby controls conscious and unconscious fears which might affect sleep. If not dealt with naturally by play, they could also cause illness. The level of the similia which she is creating must vary with each individual child – it may be concerned with birth experiences and possible unconscious traumas, or re-creating a wish to throw away the threatening new baby, or the mother who does not come immediately when needed and demanded. Most important, it allows the child to overcome blocks which could otherwise stunt development.

Drama Therapy

In Drama Therapy, it is not the patient himself who re-creates the similimum as a result of an injection or suggestion, consciously giving him 'permission' to re-create and externalize it. The patient, with the help of the drama therapist, plays or acts out in movement, shape, sound, mime, and words, the actual happenings and feelings that he was unable to contain at the time of the original stress. At that time they were swallowed up and introjected into his own psyche and his energy levels and vital resources were drained, which must inevitably limit personal relationships.

Dance Therapy is a more subtle and sophisticated form of Drama Therapy, whereby the patient re-creates the 'similimum' in the dance, perhaps not so dramatically as in abreaction – there may be no catharsis or explosion; only slowly, piece by piece. When effective, it is re-created to effect a cure.

I have mentioned Drama Therapy, and I want to recall briefly that group therapy is often part of the drama experience. In post-war office and troop rehabilitation centres, men were treated in small groups. It was not uncommon in these groups to use a combination of abreaction and drama techniques. However, frequently in the daily morning group session, helped by the group leader, intense emotion, strong feelings and fears could, and did emerge. These simulated and re-created many of the powerful parental authority-figures who played such a significant role in the background aetiology of the neurosis, and provided the 'soil', so to speak, for it.

Paranoid Personality

The paranoid personality denies the similia experience and projects outside of himself, in what may be a most terrifying and aggressive way, his 'similimum', or rather the fragments of it. It is in the fragmentation of the 'similimum' and therefore of the self – the two are inseparable – that psychosis, or a break with reality, occurs. It is these denied 'similimum' fragments which are projected out of the self, as if to surround others around him with an envelope, or aura of 'similimum' fragments, which create the severity of the illness. The 'similimum' is no longer in himself, waiting to flow out with its free vital energy and a surge of strength, but bits of the traumatic original situation are felt to be all around him. These 'similimum' fragments are watching him, influencing him, reading his mind, talking about him. Only when these fragments can be taken back into the self from their external containers and welded together inside the psyche – being accepted as part of the person, can they be exteriorized and a cure effected. Without this internalization, the result is a world of delusion, disturbance, phantasy and chaos.

Hypnosis

In Hypnosis the hypnotist may often use techniques of regression, allowing the patient to become infantile. The patient is taken back in time, if he is a suitable deep-trance subject. The aim is to recapture and recall earliest memories and events. He may be regressed year by year, birthday by birthday, and his writing and speech become progressively younger with each experience. This 'similimum' is not available to everyone, as not everyone can attain the deep-trance states. It is usually less violent than abreaction, as the patient allows the hypnotist to have a very powerful effect upon him, imposing his own calm and controls to a certain extent; never totally, however, contrary to popular belief.

Recalled early events must always be considered to be psychological 'similia' as the original hurt can never actually be recalled, however rich the detail in the regressive experience. Again this can be a very effective therapy.

Psycho-Analysis

Psycho-analysis is a very intense and prolonged two-person relationship in depth, where all aspects of the personality, and those figures which make up its configurations, emerge within the framework of the analytic relationship, to create what is usually called the 'transference'. This is regarded as a sine quae non of the curative process, enabling the patient to exteriorize both immature and mature parts of the self, however distorted, and to allow them to grow again in the soil of the psycho-analytic experience. The patient in analysis creates a whole group of 'similia' as he projects different images into the analyst from his internal world and 're-lives' those earlier experiences in the present during therapy. It is the analyst accepting the whole as part of the similimum, without criticism or judgement, which creates the cure. For very deeply disturbed personality disorders, it can be a very valuable method of growth, maturation and cure.

Similimum Principle

My reason for drawing attention to the similimum as being a basic factor in these therapies, is to suggest that a 'similimum principle' may also be an important part of our natural development and growth. We may master anxieties from childhood onwards by creating similia in our play, dreams and fantasies, as also in our relationship with others, including the vicissitudes of marriage. Mild abreaction, transference, and drama therapy may occur as part of our social interactions daily, the similimum, allowing us to work through, and overcome stress, fear, and anxiety which might otherwise become trapped, block development, with resulting symptoms and illness.

In homoeopathy we often talk and think of miasms – when well-indicated remedies fail to elicit a response. We consider them as ghosts of illnesses, and not just suppressed symptoms, involving factors inherited by other than direct chromosomal pathways – running through families from one generation to another, causing refractory patterns of illness.

This seems to happen in chronic psychological illness when there is either an inherited weakness or a family disposition towards certain patterns of illness. In these conditions the similia principle seems to be ineffective, or not to occur, and a more grave and serious illness develops which does not respond to any of the above therapies.

Unfortunately, I know of no nosode-equivalent

in modern or classical psychological techniques or therapy.

This would not, however, preclude a direct homoeopathic intervention using potentized remedies and possibly a high-potency nosode from effecting a permanent one.

However, once the normal similimum mechanism of self-defence has broken down, as outlined above, this is often a serious sign of chronic disease, and it may take many months of treatment to decide whether a response is possible and a cure obtainable.

4

Pointers to Potency

Where problems are tangible, acute and clear-cut, give the 6th centisimal potency or similar 'low' potency frequently, if necessary every few minutes until relief occurs. Where less acute – give hourly. Use a higher potency only if clearly indicated and then do not repeat so frequently as the 'low' one – but according to judgement, the individual case and responses. A 30th potency should not usually be prescribed for an acute problem unless it is the only potency available and then use hourly only. If there is little or no response with the 6c potency, change to a higher potency of the same remedy, but observe the responses to a single dose always.

Homoeopathy will not work properly if symptoms are the result of a foreign body, acute blockage, obstruction, displacement, or dislocation. These need to be adjusted, corrected and treated by a physical treatment related to their cause and the underlying problems of the patient.

As the patient improves – following an aggravation, if there is sufficient available energy, then stop the remedy and observe. In every acute case the patient is in a crisis of elimination with inability to externalize and excrete an internal irritant due to the blockage or stasis of drainage of the acute condition. Homoeopathy supports and facilitates this drainage, allowing energy flow again always provided that it is not of mechanical origin. The potency facilitates movement, energy elimination and a return to healthy functioning.

In every acute case – as throughout homoeopathy, the acute prescription should only be prescribed on the totality of individual presenting symptoms and not on pathology or a diagnostic label. Give the specific nosode once only for an acute epidemic condition when indicated or if the vital response to the indicated remedy is weak, delayed or in any way unsatisfactory.

Chronic problems – These are the most difficult of all to treat because vital response is inevitably sluggish and minimal. There is usually a long-term crisis associated with intoxication and stasis of some kind with slowing down generally of physiological responses, and failure to eliminate over a prolonged period. The body lacks the strength to achieve an acute healing aggravation or significant vital response so that there can be no resolution by the patient of blockage and stasis.

When a case is irreversible it lacks sufficient drive, vitality and energy to eliminate any internal irritating barriers and to bring them to resolution – either from physical or psychological reasons. It remains incurable and chronic within the system until a change occurs in the availability of vital response, energy and movement in the areas affected. Where the problem is irreversible, a cure left too late, the prescription should be kept to the lower 3x/6c potencies and it is an error to prescribe 'high'. High prescribing in such cases can evoke a violent reaction – even a fatal one, and is only indicated for terminal suffering, the patient dying, when it is very valuable for easing anguish, bringing peace of mind and dignity with analgesics kept to a minimum.

In chronic illness, more than with acute problems, the aim is to restore balanced vital functioning and circulation to the area – physiological and psychological responses as part of the essential responses and stimulus the patient needs. The aim is improved function and flow, overcoming of stagnation or retention with maximum stimulation of elimination and drainage which is the key to overcoming every chronic state.

Chronic problems inevitably mean blockage, failure of flow and lack of detoxication so that essential drainage is always a primal aim of the homoeopathic intervention. Once there is a return to homoeopathic aggravation, then there is equally a return to vitality and overcoming any poverty of flow or suppression of underlying dynamics. In the past there have been minor peaks or exacerbations of symptoms, but with no true aggravation and in this way the system retains its same position of stasis over prolonged periods with no real gains or vital reaction which could lead on to the resolution.

In chronic conditions a miasm must always be considered and specific anti-miasmic remedy given at an early stage in the treatment where an indicated potency fails to evoke a satisfactory response. It should not then be repeated for several months after the initial prescription and in this way resembles the nosode prescribing.

Proving the remedy – This may happen where there is sensitivity to a remedy – recurring usually only when it has been given over a prolonged period, either in low or unnecessary high potency beyond the period of symptom-recovery. If severe, the remedy should be stopped immediately and if there is no lessening of proving-symptoms, the remedy neutralized to eliminate it from the system. Such symptoms are different from a positive aggravation and it is important always to differentiate a proving sensitivity reaction from the emergence of new symptoms, or a worsening of the original condition.

An example of proving a remedy – A patient had been taking *Arnica* 6 daily on a self-prescribed basis for fatigue over several weeks. After 10 days he was considerably better but against all homoeopathic principles, he decided to continue with the remedy because he felt so well. After 3 weeks a localized intense, left-sided chest discomfort developed in the inter-costal muscles that would not go. The pain was of a severe bruised nature – as if he had been kicked. All symptoms were better for lying on the side, holding it and generally immobilizing. The bed felt unusually hard and uncomfortable. On stopping *Arnica* all symptoms disappeared within 24 hours.

5

On the Difficulties of Self-prescribing

At times, every experienced practitioner finds it necessary to prescribe for himself, or their family, especially when there is an acute condition or the usual colleague who looks after him or her is unavailable at the time. Almost invariably the homoeopath finds this difficult. Their own 'constitutional' frequently remains a mystery which they cannot easily fathom and unless they are prescribing for the most superficial first-aid condition, such as a sprain or fall, the practitioner tends to find their own prescription is ineffective or that they have got the diagnosis 'wrong' and their condition does not improve. When treating the family they are usually more successful, but even there, they are often less efficient and reliable than with their patients.

Where the causes are deeper, the problem something other than an acute or superficial problem, especially where a middle or higher potency is indicated, even the most experienced practitioner tends to be unreliable or inaccurate. The reasons are not too obscure to understand. There is often a strong emotional thread to the condition, which has undermined resistance and burned-out vitality – perhaps over a period of weeks or months, leading to a jaded psychological or physical state which is put down to 'work pressures'. This is because insight is usually lost into the true underlying mentals, or they are not admitted and looked at, denied as irrelevant – although for a patient it would have been quite different. The blockage to insight in depth, blocks accuracy of prescribing, and it is essential in homoeopathy to be able to match both the physical symptoms with the mentals for completeness and accuracy.

In some cases the remedy prescribed is correct but the potency or depth of the remedy is incorrect. Where a colleague would have taken an overall view, allowed ample time for the underlying psychologicals to emerge and taken a sensitive history, as the homoeopath would have done with his or her patients, there is often a hit and miss stab at the right remedy, from a 'hunch' or from previous 'experience', rather than from symptoms or repertorizing the clinical picture, so that a remedy is prescribed which well and truly fits the clinical facts.

Such difficulties confirm the importance of insight and understanding into the mentals and the key role they play in every case history, even the most physically presenting picture. In general it is well-known that doctors don't make good patients, even with their own family. They either struggle-on, or complain and can't easily make the shift from the caring person or active do-gooder to that of the needy, more passive needing one. Doctors also don't take kindly to accepting their own advice, which they so patiently hand out to others.

They will even not take their own medicines, which they know they need – for example to drink more fluids, or to go to bed for a couple of days. In homoeopathy especially, they rarely take the time to accurately 'take' their own case properly. What the homoeopath expects of him or herself is a quick, one-dose cure. This is not uncommon, but it is rare in self-prescribing.

Many doctors are so taken up with their practice and their patients, that they fail to admit or acknowledge that they also have a body with physical needs like everyone else, and in this way they neglect themselves over the years, often out of a sense of omnipotence or denial. Time for regular meals, for check-ups or even exercise is too often last on their list of priorities.

The working man tends to rate success in terms of a job prospering or having made money in business. When the firm is doing well he feels happy and good, when the business does badly, he is depressed. With doctors it is different, they tend more to rate themselves in terms of patient-progress. If a patient doesn't get better, the doctor gets depressed or feels a failure, if the patient is improving, then they feel 'good' and a success. This has relevance also to the doctor who is ill. He or she feels that they should not get ill and that in some way it is an admission of weakness or failure. Certainly patients don't expect their doctor to get sick – it is a music hall joke or a cause for anxiety. The doctor feels apologetic, not a good advertisement for his or her methods, and certainly nobody expects a homoeopath who knows so much and has such an impressive list of remedies to get sick. There is little sympathy for the sick doctor by the patient, in some cases by the family too. It should have been prevented and it is not a 'good' thing for the doctor or their image. A sick doctor is a nuisance, in many ways an embarrassment, certainly in hospital. Just as the patient quips 'physician heal thyself', so the doctor unconsciously sees illness as a failure and tends unconsciously to want to deny it, particularly at any early treatable stage.

Every illness has a deeper meaning to it, and often the doctor, like his patient cannot get better, until he or she is able to acknowledge the real underlying facts in themselves and is able to talk about them. Often he has been overworking, burning the candle at both ends and the illness may be felt as a punishment, judgment or consequence of his or her life not being in order, which is associated with some guilt or a feeling of neglect.

In general, doctors don't want to accept that they are vulnerable, that like their patients, they too can get ill or sick and need treatment at times, just as much and like everyone else. Perhaps they are also reluctant to think of themselves as mortal and human, thinking that they should only be a glowing example of health, wisdom, and vitality. Sometimes the doctor, like his patient needs to experience sickness, suffering and pain in order to better understand the suffering of others and to deepen his own sense of awareness, knowledge and compassion.

There is a mystique prevalent in the medical profession of immunity at all times, even in an epidemic, howevermuch repeated exposure, confidence, expertise and freedom from fear in a professional situation actually supports the development of healthy resistance. But none of us are omnipotent and when an illness 'strikes', there is a sense of having fallen from grace, of being ashamed to be 'unhealthy' and that there is a barrier to health. But illness is not something to be ashamed of, nor 'bad' in the way that the doctor sometimes feels it to be.

Illness itself offen has a message to it, which relates to the particular period of underlying need, despair or anxiety. When such needs cannot be acknowledged by the physician, they tend to be fobbed off as 'being under the weather, or tired'. In many cases the family sees more truly through the facade and can better recommend the remedy needed, more accurately than the 'patient'.

Once the doctor can accept and admit his or her own mentals, the psychological needs, which they share with everyone else, and can stop wanting to be omnipotent and immortal, seeing illness as a failure and negative, then they can also begin to better treat themselves as whole persons too, and prescribe a treatment just as effective as for their patients.

6

Holiday Remedies

Stings

Arnica is the best remedy when there is swelling, redness and discomfort, the area feeling bruised and painful. *Calendular* cream applied locally taken in the 6c potency is soothing and supports healing. Use twice daily over the area. *Ledum* is for very painful stings where the area feels chilly and cold without the sensation of heat or burning. Where a sting-reaction is of burning heat and redness, *Belladonna* is indicated. The three major remedies are *Arnica*, *Ledum* or *Belladonna* taking *Calendular* either locally or internally. *Hypericum* may be indicated for any shooting pains associated, which travel upwards along the peripheral nerves of the area, particularly in one limb.

Constipation

There are two major remedies to consider – *Nux vomica* and *Bryonia*. The difference lies in the type and degree of constipation. There are two common reasons for constipation – psychological and a change of diet. Where *Bryonia* is indicated, there is the urge to open the bowels, but nothing happens, nothing moves and when it does, the stool is small, dry, and round. *Nux vomica* has more urgent straining, with spasm or irritability and a hard painful motion. There is more movement where *Nux* is indicated and not the small, cannonball motions of *Bryonia*. The skin and whole body are dry where *Bryonia* is indicated, the stool and anal area dry from inadequate moisture to lubricate the passage of the stool. *Opium* in potency should be considered for a more chronic problem and when total, or *Aluminium* when there are also more generalized constitutional disturbances.

Diarrhoea

Diarrhoea is also common on holiday, *Arsenicum* the major remedy for both adults and children. The stool feels hot, burning and is watery when indicated. If there is sudden weakness and collapse with diarrhoea, when driving in the heat, consider *Aconitum* or *Arnica*, especially for acute or toxic conditions with shock. Follow an infective diar- rhoea – watery and offensive with *Hepar Sulph* if it does not respond to *Arsenicum* where indicated. Use *Arnica* for shock especially with infants or young children in danger of becoming dehydrated. Always hydrate a child with lots of drinks, when there has been severe diarrhoea. Hospitalization with intravenous fluid replacement may be needed in severe cases. For diarrhoea on waking without pain or spasm, associated with heat and an exces- sive fruit intake, use *Podophyllum*. In a delicate, over-sensitive disposition, with weakness and exhaustion, often after a shock or when convales- cent, use *Phosphoric ac*.

Insomnia

For not getting off to sleep, the mind over-active from worrying about tomorrow, give *Lycopodium*. When due to indigestion, with a windy indigestion, use *Carbo Veg*. When lack of sleep is due to toothache give *Chamomilla*. For sleeplessness from pain, having knocked your shin as you got out of the train or car – use *Arnica*. *Lycopodium* is for right-sided painful problems, *Kali Carb*. or *Lachesis* for left-sided ones. When there is fear and panic about travel or flying, consider *Gelsemium* or *Lycopodium*. In general *Gelsemium* is more concerned with immediate fears. *Lycopodium* has most action on anticipatory worries and future fears. Where there has been abuse of coffee or tea give *Coffea 6*.

Vomiting

For chilly diarrhoea and vomiting, but a burning stool use *Arsenicum*. For nervous vomiting, use *Gelsemium* because it has strong emotional and psychological activity. For spasms of nausea and vomiting associated with irritability, give *Nux vomica*.

Rashes

Give *Belladonna* where the skin is hot and bright red, the adult or child is restless and irritable, with loss of appetite or when sleep is disturbed. There may be a slight temperature associated, or a sore throat. Often the child is just miserable and unhappy. There may be a recurrent tendency to earache and frequent courses of antibiotics may have been prescribed. When the child is feverish, fretful and hot, or there has been a contact with measles recently, give *Belladonna*. For very acute conditions use *Aconitum*. For a more chronic problem which recurs from exposure to heat, usually with an offensive type of rash, use *Sulphur*.

Indigestion

When there has been over-indulgence with food having eaten excessively, a late evening with too much wine or coffee, bloated and restless, use *Nux vomica*. When the feelings are of restless nervousness, unable to sleep, the clock strikes one and then two, and still you cannot relax or do other than toss and turn, use *Aconitum*. For anxious indigestion and a swollen, blown-out upper abdomen with intolerance of heat, use *Argentum nitricum*.

Sunstroke and Sunburn

Having fallen asleep in the sun or over-exposed your body to the sun on the first or second day, the skin, red and hot, use *Arnica*, 6c hourly until there is relief. The main symptoms usually are of weakness, thirst, exhaustion and headache. If the skin is hot, with a restless, burning sensation of heat and a temperature, take *Belladonna*. For the ill-effects of heat of any sort with shock, use *Arnica*. For more general acute malaise with restlessness, use *Aconitum*. For the ill-effects of heat, travelling too long in the car, without shade or rest, use *Pulsatilla* for women and *Arnica* for men. Consider using 5 drops of Rescue Remedy (Bach).

Teething Problems

When a child or an adult has toothache with pain and restlessness and wants to be held or comforted, although also irritable and complaining give *Chamomilla*. Other remedies to consider are *Belladonna*, *Staphysagria* and *Nux vomica*.

Colic

For infantile, windy colic, the child doubled-up and miserable, use *Mag Phos*. For pains which cause doubling-up on the first day of a menstrual period also use *Mag Phos.*, hourly until there is relief. For colic and spasm associated with dietary over-indulgence, use *Nux vomica*. When the baby cries but is windy, doubled-up or distended, use *Carbo Veg*.

Travel Sickness

For nausea, with anxiety, dizziness, weakness or collapse, pouring out, give *Gelsemium*. This is also the remedy for an acute cold when these symptoms closely resemble those of influenza. For nausea with irritability, use *Nux vom*. For travel sickness with excessive salivation and sweating, give *Petroleum*. For nausea and travel sickness which is much more clearly emotional in origin, use *Natrum mur*.

Headache

When due to excessive exposure to the sun give *Glonoine*. For adult headache associated with dizziness or vertigo give *Gelsemium*. For sick headache following excesses of coffee or tea – *Paullinia* or *Coffea*. Where the headache is spasmodic and irritable, due to excesses of wine or food, give *Nux vomica*.

7

Remedies for the Home Medicine Chest (I)

Homoeopathy is based on two major principles. The first is concerned with a comparative study of the complaints of the patient or symptoms of the illness, which are compared with the toxic symptoms of the undiluted mother-substance used in the treatment, called the Law of Similitudes. Coffee can be used in its homoeopathic form *Coffea* for the treatment of insomnia, comparing the symptoms of the patient with the stimulating effect of coffee when taken in excess, leading to sleeplessness.

The second principle of homoeopathy which is basic to understanding, is the therapeutic usage of infinite or minimal dosages produced by successive, serial dilutions which are succussed or vitalized at each stage. This ensures safety for the patient and freedom from toxic side-effects. In this way extremely minute amounts of substances – of animal, mineral or vegetable origin – are used to make up the remedies. Such infinitesimal doses using the energy of the substance, are in harmony with the natural biological dilutions of the body, for example the extremely minute amounts of essential trace elements, such as cadmium, copper, manganese and magnesium. These are basic to cellular health, to blood and enzyme functioning and their absence causes severe disturbances, despite the minimal nature of their concentration.

Homoeopathy is above all, the science of individualization. When treating a child, the homoeopath is not concerned so much with the type of cold, but the characteristics of the child. Where there are identical twins, each one copes with and manifests the infection differently according to his or her unique and individual make-up and the homoeopath must choose the remedy most helpful for the individual child, their symptoms or reactions and temperature and not prescribe for a cold in isolation from the person. The following remedies are all basic, they should be kept at home in the 6th potency and also be taken with you on holiday.

Aconitum
This is extracted from the plant *Aconitum Napellus* (Monkshood, Hemlock). It is the most poisonous plant which grows in Europe and is found in the foothills of many European countries up to an altitude of 1,000 feet. It is a historical poison, used by both the Greeks and the Romans, and is the poison reputedly taken by Socrates. It is one of the most important of all remedies for acute conditions. A first-aid remedy, it should be used within the first 48 hours of symptoms developing. These are usually variable and occur in the throat, chest or urinary tract. Most characteristic of an *Aconitum* problem, is the excessive amount of fear and anxiety present, and to prescribe it accurately,

there should be at least some agitation or apprehension. Characteristically, the patient feels extremely ill, weak and convinced that they have a fatal condition. A young child may be screaming with fear and restlessness, the adult feels agitated and cannot relax, perhaps after a motor accident when slightly concussed or fearful after a fall from a ladder when pruning, leading to shock and agitation. They are convinced that they have a fracture or dislocated a joint, but nothing can be seen on x-ray. Despite reassurance by their doctor, they cannot sleep, and are convinced of permanent damage, that they are going to die or get worse.

It is not a remedy for the thin, but rather for those of strong stout build. A patient aged 40 was seen, an ex-Sergeant Major, of impressive stature with an enormous barrel chest, always fit, a cross-country runner and never previously ill in his life. There was an epidemic of viral influenza at the time which affected the area where he was living. He was however suddenly struck down by the infection, developing an acute viral pneumonia. Within a few hours he was in bed, with a high temperature and very agitated, convinced that this was the end. This strong, previously fit man was toppled by viral pneumonia in a few hours, and the homoeopathic remedy was undoubtedly *Aconitum*.

The *Aconitum* child is usually red-faced, chubby, agitated and tearful because of a hurting discomfort. Pain is usually present in some form as well as agitation and is the major indication for *Aconitum*. It is best used in the initial stages of an acute condition with a problem which is the outcome of fear, or when the condition is still present, ten or twenty years later, then *Aconitum* can still be indicated, provided that the initial cause was one of acute shock or fear.

Use a 30th potency when anxiety symptoms are very marked with agitation. A 6th potency is sufficient when physical symptoms predominate.

Arnica

Arnica or Fallkraut grows on the mountainous slopes of Europe. It is used in homoeopathy where the plant grows above 1,000 feet. For generations the Swiss mountain folk have taken a hot infusion for bruises, falls and sprains. It is a reliable remedy for tendon swellings, twisted ankle, or any sort of bruise, even if spontaneous, or pain which feels as though you've been kicked. It is also invaluable for fatigue, tiredness, and shock after any acute trauma.

The major mentals of *Arnica* are a crestfallen feeling. Someone says 'Can't you remember anything? What sort of person are you? Can't you do better than that?' – Where the response is a feeling of being crushed or bruised psychologically, then the remedy is *Arnica*.

Arsenicum alb

White arsenic is one of the major polycrest remedies. Polycrest means a remedy of many peaks, or actions, one which acts on general systems of the body. The indications for *Arsenicum* are a combination of exhaustion, fatigue with bowel or lung disturbance. The patient, either child or adult, is chilly, thin and usually over-active, unable to keep still. The typical *Arsenicum* temperament is perfectionistic, neat and fussy. The classic patient has been described as 'the man with a gold-headed cane'. *Arsenicum* acts strongly on the intestines, as in summer diarrhoeas, where acute liquid stools give a burning diarrhoea. Arsenic burns, but typically the patient feels a combination of feeling both chilly, weak and exhausted, yet restless with burning pains, when the remedy is indicated. It acts strongly on the chest for acute conditions and also in urinary problems. The remedy is acute, but less so than *Aconitum*. In general, it is best prescribed early, but it does not have the fear or agitation of *Aconitum* although the restlessness can be severe.

Belladonna
The toxic picture of *Belladonna*, or Deadly Nightshade poisoning is one of dilated pupils; a flushed red face; a pounding headache; a feeling of explosive burning and extreme agitation. Delirium and a high fever may be present and if you put your hand near to a patient who needs *Belladonna* you can often feel the heat. They are extremely restless and a typical clinical example where *Belladonna* is needed is the child with Otitis Media or acute middle ear infection with a high fever and an acutely painful ear. It acts strongly in this area, even when the problem is recurrent or not responding to antibiotics. It also acts strongly on an acute throat condition, providing that it feels hot, red and burning. The child may be feverish, crying, agitated and irritable. *Belladonna* is also useful for measles and it can be useful prophylactically to prevent it where there has been a contact in a weak or convalescent child.

Bryonia alb.
The wild hop-plant, common in the Kent hedgerows, has beautiful strands of white flowers.

44

Bryonia is another polycrest remedy. Its main characteristic is that any form of movement aggravates the symptoms. Where a child has a cough, it is worsened by movement. It is a strong remedy for the chest, and in pleurisy, the side is held to 'fix' the chest and to lessen the pain of movement and coughing. The classic *Bryonia* comment is 'Don't move me, don't push me, don't touch me!' It affects the whole body, but especially the lung pleural cavity lining layers and the joints where it rivals *Rhus tox* for painful conditions, worse for walking, exercise, or climbing stairs.

The typical *Bryonia* mentals are a state of irritability. Dryness is characteristic, even of the humour and temperament. The throat, skin and mucous membranes are dry, with all secretions the chalky-white colour of wild flower. There is clear phlegm, clear mucous nasal discharge but the tongue has the typical white coating.

8

Remedies for the Home Medicine Chest (II)

Carbo Veg

Carbo Veg is made from vegetable charcoal and has been used since antiquity as a body cleanser and purifier. The typical mentals of the remedy are sluggishness. The mind is sluggish, as much as the circulation. Everything is slow, indolent, lazy and inert, almost to the point of appearing stupid. A patient has fainted, lies lifeless, marble-like, cold and covered with sweat. They can't move, are without energy and look as if they are dying. This inability to express, with lack of strength or will-power and feeling at death's door is typical. It is a great reviver *par excellence*, the *Carbo Veg* person sluggish, puffy and largely immobile. Flatulence is a major indication for the remedy and it is common to find most distension in the upper abdomen. It is excellent for both a sluggish intestinal condition as well as for problems of poor circulation such as varicose veins. It is also useful in more chronic conditions such as leg varicose ulcers, bed sores and generally unhealthy areas of skin particularly of the elderly. It is not a remedy however which is associated with much pain.

Chamomilla

The tincture of the whole *Chamomilla* plant, was used on lawns in Elizabethan times and in their herbal gardens. *Chamomilla* is a well-known remedy for teething problems of childhood and helpful for painful gums, but it is also useful in many adult conditions. The key notes are of pain that seems beyond endurance associated with considerable irritability. The *Chamomilla* child with teething problems won't lie down, wants to be held and screams, kicks, or gets into a fury when put down. The adult who needs *Chamomilla* is also worse for rest and for lying down. There is a need for movement and a similar pattern of anger and irritation as in the child. The man with a *Chamomilla* backache, has intolerable pain and is irritable. The woman with *Chamomilla* menstrual colic is also irritable and worse for rest or lying down. The anger and restlessness are usually worse in the evening. *Chamomilla* should always be considered for any intolerable pain with irritability and where bed-rest or lying down aggravates the problem. This is a paradoxical situation with a painful condition, worse for rest rather than relieved by it. Sullen anger, refusal to speak, a wilful child, resentful at being touched, resentment at questions are all typical of *Chamomilla* being indicated.

Gelsemium semperiens

Tincture of the root and bark of the yellow Jasmine plant is used as an important remedy for weakness and 'flu'-like conditions. The typical *Gelsemium* mood is one of fright, fear and anxiety. It is a remedy used for decades by homoeopaths for examination 'funk' as it used to be called. Fear, anticipation, hysteria, 'nerves', especially where the person feels they cannot cope or are going to be inadequate. There is a conviction of failure with terror, or stage fright. *Gelsemium* has healing potential for shivery, cold, weak, acute conditions. There may be a chill, but it is also helpful in pre-menstrual problems when it is less marked. Typical symptoms are a cold, shivery, weakened, anxious condition. It is a remedy for weakness and paralysis in other areas and it is also one of the few remedies where anticipatory anxiety leads to diarrhoea. The nervous child has an 'accident' but not one of the bladder, always of the bowels. Diarrhoea with associated fear is an indication, also paralysis or a weight-like sensation in the legs – typical of acute 'flu'. It is not a remedy for a major influenza epidemic when the nosode *Influenzinum* or *Aconitum* may be more indicated. But for viral colds which everyone calls 'flu', *Gelsemium* is invaluable. Anxiety and fearfulness are the typical mentals and these are usually present in some form where it is indicated.

Hepar Sulph.
Hepar Sulph. is an interesting remedy made up of equal parts of the scrapings of the inner oyster shell and flowers of sulphur. It is an ancient remedy and has been used over the centuries for chronic skin problems and gout in particular.

The mentals are irritability, anger, impulsiveness, dissatisfaction, nervous dejection, but particularly cross irritability, peevishness, and oversensitiveness are the keynote. The flowers of sulphur aspect has a value for puffy infections, inflammation, skin eruptions or ear infection without the high temperature that is more typical of *Belladonna*. Chronic ear and throat infections, tonsillitis, local inflammation, ulceration, offensive discharges may all indicate *Hepar Sulph*. Interestingly, it is said that they take a lot of vinegar when they eat their chips and pour it on, which seems to indicate a preference for sour, acidy foods.

Hypericum

Tincture of the whole St Johns Wort plant is used for one of the major remedies in homoeopathy.

The mentals are fear, restlessness and nervous depression. It is used for nerve tissue damage and small, localized puncture wounds. *Arnica* is for soft tissue damage, *Rhus Tox* is for muscle damage, *Symphytum* is for bone damage, but *Hypericum* is for damage to any area with a rich supply of nerves. A kick on the shin or periosteol membrane bone covering hurts because there is no protection for the nerve supply there. Typical symptoms are shooting pains going up the limb, bruising, swelling, and a sticking, darting, jumping, knife-like pain shooting upwards. It is an early, acute remedy for any puncture bite from a small animal. The damaged area is usually red, inflamed and tender, the skin broken. It may be infected with swelling or obstruction in the area. Nervous anxiety and restlessness combined with wound damage to nervous tissue and shooting pains strongly indicates *Hypericum*.

9

Remedies for the Home Medicine Chest (III)

Kali Bic
Potassium Bicromate is one of the major remedies in homoeopathy and it is needed in every home remedy box. It is a remedy where the mentals are not particular indicated, acting predominantly on the mucous membrane which begins at the lips and ears, anal and genital areas and lines the essential body organs. Symptoms initially are of an outpouring of clear fluid or mucous. An itchy irritation may develop, becoming thick and yellow. If you think of the nasal mucous, when a typical catarrhal condition is most obvious, this gives the typical picture of *Kali bic* with a thick, yellowy discharge. It is the family remedy for all irritating congestions of mucous membrane. It is not the only remedy that acts in that area – *Pulsatilla* is also effective in sinus and mucosal problems but lacks the specificity of *Kali bic*. It is a useful remedy for ear and nasal congestion, also of any part of the mucous membrane, including vaginal discharges. Thickening of the membrane occurs due to congestion and this can be from any cause – infection, allergy or irritation,

but in homoeopathy, the cause is always secondary to the individual symptoms. The other area where *Kali bic* is useful is in stomach complaints. A common cause of indigestion is congestion of the stomach mucosal lining, causing gastric upsets in adults or children. It is also useful for peptic ulceration. A patient was run down and at a low ebb, with multiple ulcers around the gum area. *Kali bic* was the indicated remedy and the condition was cured after a mild initial aggravation of the condition.

Ledum

Another local remedy is *Ledum*, or Marsh Tea. It is a remedy for penetrating wounds, rather resembling *Hypericum*'s action on nervous tissue. A remedy for the child that crushes a finger in the door, it also helps with splinters, or any wound from treading on a pin, needle or a nail. The main characteristic of a *Ledum* wound is the absence of any heat and a cold sensation in the area affected. This is not a *Belladonna* reaction of heat, or an *Arsenicum* response of burning. There may be a foreign body present – which needs removing, or a clean, penetrating wound with stinging pain and chilliness. The person feels cold, the area chilled or cool. All symptoms are in general better for cold. It seems paradoxical that they want to be cool, even though the area affected may be quite cold.

Lycopodium

Lycopodium, or Club Moss is one of the most important remedies in the repertory. It is a polycrest remedy of general action throughout the body and cellular system, and fully worthy of study. Its period of action is from six to eight weeks when taken and it is often prescribed 'high' in a single remedy dose. It acts particularly on the right-side of the body – a right-sided nasal blockage, a right-sided throat condition, or a chest condition. It also acts on the bladder – not on the right side but it could do. It will also act on right-sided wounds or bruises. It is also associated with dryness of the skin where sweating is minimal. All symptoms are worse in the late afternoon to early evening, about 4–8.00 p.m. A child with a right-sided throat, nasal blockage, or earache without the high temperature of *Belladonna*, and less acute than where *Aconitum* is indicated, responds well to *Lycopodium*. It is useful for insomnia and helpful for relaxation, anxiety, examination 'nerves' or stage fright. The other remedy for examination nerves is *Gelsemium*. *Lycopodium* often follows *Gelsemium* in anxiety problems of the child or adult who is a worrier and crosses bridges before they come to them.

Magnesium Phosphate
This is another local remedy, almost a homoeopathic aspirin, for colicky neuralgic pains, better for heat, movement, and for doubling-up. It is a useful remedy for spasmodic period pains, relieved by warmth, pressure and moving around.

Natrum Mur
Many homoeopaths would agree that if they had to choose only one remedy to work with, it would be either *Lycopodium* or *Natrum Mur*. I would possibly opt for *Natrum Mur* or *Arnica*, if limited to the single remedy. Common salt in potency, it is a polycrest working on the whole body. Acting deeply at cellular level it is not markedly right or

left sided in action. The characteristic mentals are anxiety, restlessness and a desire to be alone. *Lycopodium* wants to be alone but prefers someone else in the house because they are insecure. *Natrum Mur* just wants to be alone because others aggravate them. They do not need a shoulder to cry on and dislike company and the demands of others. It acts on mucous membrane like *Kali bic* but deeper and more widely. A key point is that the eyes water in the wind and with laughter. It is good for chronic problems and for obscure non-specific 'difficult' problems. It acts powerfully on the urinary system and symptoms are better for local pressure. A typical example is *Natrum Mur* backache which is improved by firm local pressure. They are aggravated by the sea air and tend to crave salt. Excessive salt intake with meals is often the key to the underlying pathology. They have taken so much salt that the body cannot absorb any more and this is usually the underlying cause of any disease. There is hardening of tissues – the lens (cataract), the circular muscular fibres of the arteries (arterio-sclerosis). When *Natrum Mur* is indicated, the tissues in general are tough and firm without softness or often swollen and bloated from water retention.

10

Remedies for the Home Medicine Chest (IV)

Nux Vomica

Nux Vomica is an extract of the strychnine nut and one of the most important of all the homoeopathic remedies. If you have ever read about strychnine poisoning in a novel, you will know the mortifying effects of strychnine. They are not far removed from rigor mortis itself, and an overdose of strychnine causes the most acute, painful contraction of muscles. The face grimaces, the body bends backwards and everything is in spasm. Homoeopathic strychnine is also a powerful homoeopathic remedy for spasm in any area of the body including the eye, although not specific for that area. In homoeopathy we always carefully consider the mental picture of the patient to have some insight into the underlying psychological manifestations of the person. Whenever *Nux Vomica* is indicated, there is spasm of the psychological aspects, usually expressed as irritability. Irritability of muscles is felt as spasm, cramp or pain. Spasm of the muscles of the stomach wall causes gastric cramp. If there is a problem of irritability, associated with constipa-

54

tion, cramp or spasm, the remedy is often *Nux Vomica*. The typical personality is one vulnerable to the stress diseases of civilization. They are over-competitive people, as well as irritable and driving. Energy levels are high and they are achievers. They succeed but at a cost to themselves and also to those around them. If they do not succeed, they feel a failure and so success is an all or nothing matter. Unable to delegate because they dislike relying on others, they take on too much, work at home and weekends and are in a high coronary risk group. Coronary spasm is a not uncommon warning for them to slow down.

A patient came with pain in the chest aggravated by hurrying and chill. It was not however typical angina pain, due to constriction of the coronary vessels, but there was spasm which suggested *Nux Vomica* as a remedy. For *Nux* to be well-indicated, irritability is nearly always present, and the patient often loses control of their temper and then feels guilty about it. But the next day in spite of all good intentions, the pressure builds up and it may happen again.

Phosphorus
There is a marvellous image of *Phosphorus*, quite easy to recall, where the person is drawn like a Swan Vesta match. The *Phosphorus* patient is like the stem of the match, slim, underbuilt and very vulnerable in both body and in mind. The chest is weak and respiratory infection or asthma are common. The belly is weak as in *Nux*, but with *Phosphorus* everything goes to the chest. There is cough, wheezy breathing or shortness of breath. Most symptoms concerned with *Phosphorus* as in phosphorus poisoning are linked to burning. There

are burning pains, and like the match they flare up or flush with a burning redness. Blushing, circulatory instability, redness of the neck and heat spasms are common, as are burning pains, burning diarrhoea or a burning cough. The psychological aspects are nearly always lack of confidence with anxiety. Dr. Blackie always used to say that a *Phosphorus* patient never takes their eyes off you, watching with a kind of fearfulness. The paradox about *Phosphorus* is that there are burning pains, but they crave ice-cold drinks, although chilly and feel much better for cold drinks. It is this thin, anxious, tall person, with a weak chest and sudden flashes of burning pain or burning diarrhoea who most accurately reflects the profile of the remedy.

Sulphur
Another burning remedy is *Sulphur*. Think of brimstone, sulphur, and Hades to capture the typical symptoms. *Sulphur* fumes and bubbles, with offensive discharges, nausea and burning pains. *Phosphorus* carries no fat and is always chilly, with no physiological vest. *Sulphur* is always well-layered, round, well-proportioned and warm-blooded. Warm on the coldest days, they rarely feel the cold. Offensive, irritating discharges are typical. It is a useful remedy for skin complaints. Where *Nux Vomica* is an intestine remedy, *Phosphorus* a chest medicine, *Sulphur* acts strongly on the skin. It also acts on every organ of the body. All symptoms are worse for either washing, or the application of water. Where there is a stomach or intestinal problem, there are also noisy bubbling symptoms. The breath or the burping is offensive, often there is pus and the problem is usually a chronic one. The psychological aspects of *Sulphur*

are being laid back on reality. All plans are for tomorrow with every action put off until a later date. Full of unreal ideas, they are great talkers but not good achievers. The *Nux Vomica* patient is an achiever, but at a price. *Sulphur* patients are unreal optimists. One day it will all come together and happen, but there are no plans made, no decisions taken, at least not in the foreseeable future. They have a plan, an ideal, but nothing based on reality. Everything is wonderful, even rubbish is wonderful, as long as it entails no action and no commitment. Bubbling along in a fantasy world, there is a mixture of unreality and chronic infective problems, which like the ideas, never fully resolve or come to anything.

Sepia

The potentized ink of the cuttle fish, it is a cold fish remedy for the slim, thin, irritable and often very angry individual. When first proven, Hahnemann was working in Paris and called to see an artist with the severe dragging down abdominal pains. He was sucking his brush when painting with sepia colour and this gave Hahnemann the clue to using *Sepia* as a remedy. Pain in the low back, abdomen and uterus are common, especially in a 'difficult', tired, or exhausted person. Everything is an effort. It is a unique remedy for depression. The psychological aspects of *Sepia* are extreme irritability, exhaustion and tiredness, worse in the evening and a general negative attitude. Whatever you say is wrong, or causes irritation, however helpful you try to be. 'Leave me alone, why do you keep talking? or why don't you say something?' is typical. Defeating and defeatist, they feel miserable, depressed and hopeless. The indications are dragging-down pains in any part of the body – low back, tummy or uterus, worn out, with no energy. It is primarily a female remedy but it is also of value in the male. It is a common mistake to only think of *Nux Vomica* as a male remedy, that *Sepia* is a female remedy and *Chamomilla* is only indicated for children. *Sepia* is often cold, constipated and so worn out that they just cannot get on top of their fatigue. They are off everything – family, sex, children and food. Nothing is right, nothing pleases.

Thuja

The tree of life remedy is for chronic problems like *Sulphur*, but without the burning symptoms. Indicated for dark, oily-skinned, thin and chilly people, it is useful in any condition which followed an adverse vaccination reaction. It also relieves any ill-effects of tea drinking. Many people drink tea all day long, cup after cup. *Thuja* is associated with pale, flaccid people, without much energy, generally unwell and unhealthy, who have an upset gastric or bowel condition. The other great indication is warts, particularly of the cauliflower type. These are often large with a thin stalk or root to them. They can occur in various areas of the body, especially on the foot, or the anal and genital areas. *Thuja* is an excellent remedy for these rough-headed warts and they are a major indication for *Thuja*. The many psychologicals are depression without marked irritability, and general despondency.

11

A Proving of Kali Carb

A proving of Kali Carb. was carried out in London from April 23 to June 20, 1978. Nine volunteers took part in a double blind study. Placebo in the form of Sac. Lac. tablets was given to three of the volunteers, chosen by random selection.

Kali Carb. was given to the other six provers twice daily, in tablet form during three separate terms of two weeks, in ascending potency, beginning with the 6c, followed by a break of a week without proving. Kali Carb. 30c was then taken twice daily for two weeks. After a further gap of a week, between the potencies, the 200c form was given for a final two week period.

The Provings

Each volunteer was given a diary, which was organized under headings – beginning with the mentals and then listing the principal physiological areas of the body, to be recorded on a daily basis.

Provers were all interviewed weekly during the whole of the experimental period. Their general health and diary was discussed, to ensure clarity and accuracy of recording and the presence of modalities when present. We had started with a total of eleven provers initially, but unfortunately the two youngest provers failed to keep their diaries in detail and were reluctant to attend for weekly discussion meetings, the only apparent reason for them not completing the required period of the experiment.

The Proving of Kali Carb. and Main Site of Action

Both mental and physical symptoms were well-marked. The mental symptoms were present from the second day of proving, increasing in intensity as the experiment progressed, and as an increasingly higher potency was given. The most marked mental symptoms were listlessness, fatigue, lack of energy and depression.

Throat and nasal areas of the body were consistently affected in all the provers without exception – mainly catarrhal symptoms, particularly of the left nostril, with a clear yellow discharge; itching and sneezing, and a dry sore throat. Three of the provers developed Hay fever and the symptoms were linked with the pollen count. Severe Hay fever was present in three of the provers on the lowest pollen count recording of the year.

The Bronchial passages were affected, with dry cough in three of the provers, and one prover developed severe bronchospasm – after a clear period of fifteen years without asthma symptoms.

Constipation was present in three of the provers – indicating sluggish action and inactivity of the large bowel – this was most marked in the 6c potency, the stools being small, round, hard balls of faeces.

A further marked area of action was pain in the large joints of the body, particularly the elbow and knee – on the left side of the body.

Insomnia was present in three of the six provers in the 30c potency.

The Modalities

Most of the symptoms were worse on waking, and again in the late evening about 10 p.m. The symptoms of depression and fatigue were often better in the afternoon, but endogenous in type, by being consistently worse on waking and in the morning. Nasal and throat symptoms were marked in all the provers, usually worse in the morning at 7.00 a.m. and in the evening at 6.00 p.m. and 10.00 p.m. The symptoms were worse in the left nostril and in a centrally heated room, better for fresh air. Cough, initially dry and then productive of green yellow sputum – was again worse on waking and in the late evening, worse for a dry and dusty atmosphere, better for drinking. Hay fever symptoms were marked and severe, generally worse on waking and in the evening, better for physical exercise and fresh air. Back and limb pains – were almost consistently large joint and left-sided, better for rest, worse for sitting, < fatigue, < cold, worse on waking and in the evening, better for rest.

Discussion and Summary

The symptoms of Kali Carb. evoked by the provings fall largely into the recorded materia-medica picture of the remedy.

Lassitude, weakness, fatigue, lack of energy, feeling tired and sleepy during the day, and depression were marked features of the proving. This weakness which is so characteristic of a Potassium-ion imbalance is referred to in all the classical accounts of Kali Carb. The characteristic swelling and oedema of the upper lids was seen, as also flatulence after meals, asthma, and limb pains – in particular of the knees, elbows and low back. Constipation was a feature. However there were certain differences, contrasting with earlier writings. The time modalities were worse in the morning on waking and worse in the evening.

Kali Carb. has always been described as affecting the right side of the body, and not as a left-sided remedy, which was so marked in this proving. The patients are usually stated to be intolerant of touch – but this was not a feature in the symptom-picture, nor was there any marked pre-menstrual aggravation as described by Allen in his keynotes. Nash describes amelioration of the asthma by sitting-up and rocking – but this again was not a feature. The pains in the limbs were rather vague, fleeting and non-specific rather than having a stitch-like or tearing quality – as described by Nash and Clarke. Dryness is usually considered to be a feature of the remedy. Nash compares the stitching pains with *Bryonia* – which has very marked dryness in all its symtomatology, but in the proving, the cough was dry at times, also the mouth but also often moist and productive. The skin tended to be greasy and fragile rather than dry.

References

ALLEN, T. A. – Vol. V Encyclopaedia of Pura Materia Medica. Boericke & Tafel 1877.
HAHNEMANN, S. – Chronic Diseases Vol. IV Ballere 1846.

GIBSON – British Homoeopathic Journal Vol. LIV No. 2, April 1965.

LATHOUD – Etudes de Matiere Medicale Homoeopathique Vol. 2.

FARRINGTON, E. A. (MD) – Comparison in Materia Medica with Therapeutic Hints p. 268. Dr A. Bagchi, Calcutta.

ALLEN, H. C. – Keynotes and Characteristics with Comparisons of some of the Leading Remedies of the Materia Medica. Boericke & Tafel 1916.

NASH, E. B. – Leaders in Homoeopathic Therapeutics. Nat. Homoeo. Lab. Calcutta. 1962.

CLARKE, J. H. – A Dictionary of Practical Materia Medica Vol. II Hom. Pub. Co. London, 1925.

Kali Carb. Proving – Comprehensive Summary

The provings were carried out from April 23 to June 20, 1978. There were 6 provers and three controls. The potencies were 6c, 30c and 200c.

Mind Tired, concentration difficult, restless, < evening 6.00–10.00 p.m. Tearful, not sleeping well, listless, no energy, depressed, sleepy during the day, worried, mood changes, swings from being elated, optimistic, irritable, exhausted, feeling of slight nausea, anxious, not capable of sustained mental effort, loss of confidence, lethargic, sluggish, bored, less tactful with people and more hasty with decision making, despondence, wants to be alone, fatigued, lassitude, < standing; > sitting, drained – physically and mentally.

Head Headache < evening, headache behind eyes, head feels heavy, feeling faint, headache left frontal region.

Eyes Itching, over-sensitive to light, right eye painful, eyes heavy, upper lids puffy.

Ears Coldness sensation in left ear.

Nose Slight clear to yellow discharge, itching, blocked on one side, catarrh > open air, > activity; sneezing, < in evening; thin clear discharge left nostril, stuffed with catarrh; both nostrils blocked, < evening and morning, left nostril blocked on waking, sneezing, hay fever, clear discharge all day, < morning, evening, and when yawning, sneezing, < out of doors; coryza, or common cold symptoms.

Teeth Painful near gums; gums bleed easily.

Mouth Sore, dirty taste, dry, roof of mouth itching > drinking. Cold sore on upper and lower lip. Upper lips puffy, painful.

Throat Slightly sore, tickle on retiring, < opening mouth, < yawning on waking and in evening, irritated, > hot drink. Phlegm in throat, feeling as if it needs clearing, burning, slight laryngitis > after talking > evening. Nasal voice, dry and sore.

Appetite Either loss, or increased, nausea after eating, variable and muddled. Wants to eat when not hungry. Desires salt and sweets.

Thirst Thirst for hot drinks, increased thirst.

Abdomen Slight bloated feeling, nausea, regurgitation of acid, heart-burn, 'hot bubble' sensation, < mid-day, vomited on rising, nausea of waking, distended feeling, pain, acid-taste < on lying down, nausea in evening, wind (anal), distended after meals, colicky pains < 1.30 a.m., windy indigestion, 'chest feels full of wind'.

Stool and Anus Alternating diarrhoea and constipation, urgent need to pass frequent stool. Constipation, faeces round hard balls.

Urinary Frequency during the day, dribbles after passing urine.

Sexuality Male – less libidinal drive. Female periods heavier than usual.

Chest Bronchospasm on retiring; cough with small amount of phlegm, < 8.00 a.m.–10.00 p.m., < dry atmosphere, dust, > drinking cold water; tight, raw hacking dry cough as if foreign body in throat, white sputum, < evening, > out-of-doors; yellow sputum in morning, not > for steam inhalation. Upper chest sore; bronchospasm on waking; bronchospasm during night, woke from sleep – 4.00 a.m., intermittent cough during day.

Limbs Generally tired.

Upper limbs Ache left elbow; left fingers ache; aching left shoulder and left forearm.

Lower limbs Pain left knee, < exercise; stiff hip on waking; > rest, ache left low back, < carrying, > heat.

Generalities Fatigue, accident prone, chilly, giddy, sensitive to light, intolerant of heat, clumsy.

Skin More fragile and easily damaged, greasy on forehead and nose.

Sleep Poor, disturbed, waking 4.00 a.m., restless, heavy, seems inadequate, wakes with nasal catarrh, thirsts for water in night, tired on waking, not sleeping well, wakes hourly with wind and cramp, uncomfortable lying left side, better sleeping right side.

12

Noises that Make You Sick

Low frequency pollution or 'hum' is now recognized as a major health hazard for many people, adding to the numerous environmental factors affecting the quality of life. Sensitivity to low frequency atmospheric noise has been known about for twenty-five years but it came more to the fore in the 60s and 70s when there were increasing complaints and cases of ill-health directly due to it. On the other hand, the dangers of high-pitch, high frequency noise have been known for many years. Deafness and auditory nerve damage as a result of repeated exposure to gun noise is well documented. And now, damage from disco noise is to some extent in the public eye as a potential danger.

But low frequency noise hazards are less well documented. It is likely that there are many sufferers who do not associate their symptoms with such environmental pollution so the cases are never reported. In 1977, however, an article in a national paper prompted over 750 letters from people with experience of it. This sparked off a campaign of research and fact-finding which is still in process.

The problem affects every area of the country and every age group. It is usually described as sensitivity and irritation to a low-pitch, industrial or transport noise which resembles a diesel motor idling. The pitch is variable but most commonly it is between 20–50 Hz and often only just audible. Symptoms are numerous but usually include such difficulties as restless insomnia, giddiness, a sense of fullness or vibration in the head, stress pains of the neck and ears, sometimes involving the arms or legs. Indigestion may be present.

In 1980 Walford described the problem in a paper, relating it closely to tinnitus, although it is now known that it is quite separate in most cases. Other causes of hum which need to be differentiated are those of venous or vascular origin, particularly noticeable in the quiet of the early hours, and hums due to the electro-magnetic field acting on dental fillings. The latter occurs close to the source of the noise, whereas, with low frequency hum, the source may be at a distance of a quarter of a mile or more.

The subject has been raised at a conference of The National Society for Clean Air and Chelsea College in London has developed a research programme to explore the extent of the problem.

In most cases of noise irritation, the body has the ability to adapt and neutralize or lessen its effect with time. But a major factor with low frequency hum is that the body is often quite unable to adjust to it through use. On the contrary, the symptoms intensify so the problem increases with time and the loudness and irritation seem to grow.

Not everyone is sensitive to it. Individual reaction may, however, be related to the particular pitch of the sound and a varying, pulsating pattern, accounting for the acute irritation and disturbance, particularly the absence of any balancing high wave frequency sounds of the 2000 Hz level and above to offset its intensity and continued drone. Compressors, generators, pumps, combustion engines and industrial noises are the commonest sources.

Case History

A woman of 60 came with a problem of generalized headaches and insomnia since being exposed in her home to low frequency noise from a large industrial cold store completed in 1977 about a quarter of a mile from her house. The noise from its generator could be clearly heard intermittently through the double glazing every hour of the day and night. She was also sensitive as a result of exposure to a source of low frequency noise in another town some ten miles away where at least two or three times a week she visited a relative dependent upon her. She associated the source of the second hum with a vibration in the conduits of natural gas which was being piped through close by. The symptoms from this area of exposure were slightly different, with greater loss of concentration, a varying degree of left eye pain and deterioration of vision on the same side.

A homoeopathic pharmacist made up for her a homoeopathic potency of the low frequency noise by exposing a 50% ethanol-water mixture to the vibrations in each area for forty-eight hours. It was then made up into the 6th centesimal potency and given to the patient three times daily in tablet form. Note that the potency was her specific environmental low frequency noise, rather than low frequency hum generally which could also have been potentized but with less specificity.

The results were rapid and startling. The patient telephoned me after a fortnight to say how much better she felt already both at home and at her relative's by taking the specific potency for each environmental area which I had labelled for her. There was a rapid lessening of the headaches as well as improved sleeping and a greater feeling of relaxation and contentment in the home. After a further two weeks, practically all the symptoms had completely gone and she was forgetting to take her potency – and to think about the hum which had troubled her for so long. In the area she regularly visited, she was also far better and the symptoms had disappeared. Her concentration particularly in that environment improved markedly. When there was a tendency for slight symptoms to return in the area, these were rapidly relieved by taking one tablet only of the specific potency.

The reader may wonder if this is indeed a homoeopathic achievement or merely the result of placebo or suggestion. In general, placebo results quickly wear off after ten to fourteen days; also, suggestion rarely reaches the depths of symptom-disturbance which this patient had and with such consistency.

Of course one cannot argue or deduce too much from one case but it does suggest that homoeopathy is an environmental medicine of the first order and that its results can be as consistent and outstanding as they are in many other fields. The specificity of homoeopathy for each patient is well illustrated by this particular problem and shows how it can be applied to very varied problems due to the flexibility of approach and the dynamizing of an exposed solution by the homoeopathic potency method.

It is hoped that homoeopathy will develop much more in this important field. It can and should be used to complement other attempts to clean up the environment, with homoeopathy perhaps setting the example of how a simple and natural approach can be just as effective as a sophisticated, chemical one – in some cases, even more so.

13

Insomnia

Sleep is such a precious gift that we all take for granted. It is all too easily lost or undermined by physical or psychological causes and sometimes the whole sleep-pattern may be lost for months or years.

The young baby sleeps for almost 24 hours a day, apart from hunger-pang times, and only slowly becomes more alert and aware, sleeping less, unless the birth process itself has been unduly traumatic and mechanical leading to some degree of subtle brain damage so that the whole pattern of rest and activity is interfered with from the earliest time and sleep is never full and natural from birth onwards.

The older the person, the less sleep in needed. There are many exceptions but, often with age, 5–6 hours a night seems to be enough; although, like the young child, the elderly can also cat-nap after lunch to make up the proverbial eight hours.

Sleep varies with solar seasons and the equinox as much as with our own seasons and there is quite a natural tendency in everyone to wake early in summer and to sleep on in the winter months which is unrelated to light, the dawn chorus or

British Summer Time. These patterns and physiological clocks are some of our most sensitive areas and easily upset by rapid travel. Time bands and jet-lag can upset the most inveterate and regular sleeper for periods of up to a week or more in some cases, especially where the journey has been against the sun, travelling from West to East.

The adolescent can easily sleep through until 10 or 11 a.m. at any time of the year, or be up at 4 a.m. for a fishing trip or start of the family holiday. Up and active into the early hours at a gig or disco party, they can be quite exhausted during the school term by 8 p.m. Again at weekends the teenager can be energetic and wide awake at 11 p.m. listening to music, top of the pops or the late TV film.

Adult sleep need varies as much as individual temperament. For the healthy adult, without any excessive stress or pressures, 6–8 hours a night is enough, according to need and activity. Only the shift-worker, the night nurse, ship-builder, miner, factory-floor assembler with a varying on and off night-timetable can at times have chronic, intractable insomnia problems due to work's changing patterns, yet on holiday sleep soundly as soon as they have adjusted and broken with the habit of cat-napping throughout the day and being wide-awake at night.

The causes of sleeplessness are disturbance within the three basic levels of man himself. There is a physical cause, particularly where pain and discomfort in a variety of ways causes interference with the sleep rhythms. It is the most acute in many ways with marked tension and spasm. The psychological is perhaps the most common cause of all and anxiety, depression, tension, fear are at a high level. Not uncommonly the symptoms are either aggravated or perpetuated by the variety of tranquillizers or sedatives that are prescribed with all the risks of dependency, side-effect and aggravation of the problem. The third cause is at the deepest inspirational-existential layer of man where the undermining factor is neither physical nor psychological but one of anguish.

Sleep is not only taken for granted but it is also one of man's most abused gifts. This abuse happens at every age and when continued can quickly and permanently undermine sleep. Excesses tumble resistance to zero with over-tiredness becoming a problem so that a whole range of difficulties and problems may start to appear. There is only one area of man that is more vulnerable to abuse than sleep and that is peace of mind. Unfortunately both are abused and taken for granted – at expensive cost to the individual and often to the nation as a whole.

Case History

A girl of eleven came today with a three-year history of migraines. Apart from being over-sensitive, there were no obvious psychological factors to account for her problems. There had been no fall, no family influences or pressures or identifications and no organic illness. The only other symptom was that she was over-weight for her age and height. The cause of the migraines went back to a time when there had been a marked abuse of the sleep pattern over a prolonged period because children were staying at the house and she had gone to bed late, yet was up at 6 a.m. to groom and exercise the pony. The combination of fatigue in an excitable-sensitive, energetic temperament had triggered-off a pattern of migraine that by the age of eleven was almost chronic and intractable. Snacking on sweet biscuits had also dated since that time and accounted for the weight factor. It was part of an overall problem of over-activity and disturbance since the period of sleep abuse.

Physical Causes

This is the most superficial layer with acute, often recent, physical symptoms, where restlessness, tension, agitation and secondary anxiety may be present.

The causes are many and vary from the pain of arthritis, lumbago, sciatica, indigestion or vertigo in the adult to teething problems in the young baby, the acute ear infection of the child or sudden throat or tonsillar problem with screaming acute pains, temperature, restlessness and insomnia. Asthma may be a problem at any age from childhood onwards, sometimes complicating either chronic hay-fever, bronchitis, chronic eczema, or problems of sinus or nasal congestion – any of the above suddenly increasing in severity can act as a trigger and background to the acute asthma attack, often in the middle of the night and needing help and support, sometimes hospitalization, if very acute.

Other physical causes for insomnia and broken sleep are hunger in the young baby, waking the parents for breast or bottle, with windy indigestion or colic which interferes with essential infant sleep and preventing rest and comfort. This is a time when the parents can also get over-fatigued. When there is a second young child, the fatigue of the first may be barely recovered from – where the gap is short and both or either parent can easily and quickly become over-tired and unable to sleep because of the infant demands.

A brain-damaged overactive, restless, whimpering or moaning child is a special problem, usually sleeping lightly, with no real or true sleep pattern ever properly established. The problem may have occurred after a precipitate, traumatic birth or one where instruments were necessary. There may also have been no clear-cut history for the child's hyper-activity and the light sleeping and wakefulness seems to be a continuation of day-time restlessness and overactivity: at best up and down, sleeping lightly, easily crying or calling and somehow never properly and deeply asleep – causing havoc and agonizing with the parents' own sleep and rest patterns.

There are no aspirins or pain-killers as such in homoeopathy and where pain is deep-seated and unbearable, conventional remedies must be resorted to with homoeopathy playing a secondary supportive role, but always enhancing their action and reducing ultimately the amount needed.

When there is a cancer problem with pain constant and chronic then the correct homoeopathic remedy in the right potency gives serenity and peace of mind and lessens the amount of opiates needed. Physical problems, especially the long Indian summer of '83, breaking all records, has been a severe problem for many with insomnia provoked by high city temperatures in the 80s at night.

Many have loved the heat of '83 and, with their rheumatic and rheumatoid conditions never better, have slept soundly throughout. But others have suffered and been restless, too hot, flinging the bedclothes off as stifling, yet just as quickly too chilly; up and down, fidgety, unable to settle, sleep or rest – a disturbance to themselves and all around them as they complain about the airless atmosphere and the heat.

Diarrhoea and menstrual colic are some of the other problems which may intrude or undermine sleep at this level. Insomnia can also be a side-effect of certain drug-treatments where the insomnia, the restlessness and malaise, are a complication of physiological upset from the drugs, particularly the psychotrophic groups of synthetics.

Psychological Causes

These may result from a variety of combinations of temperament, comment, personality clashes, people and demands generally. The problem usually centres around a relationship which is not going according to plan and expectation. All too often there has been a clash of temperament, perhaps not declared at the time but later leading to tears and troubled sleep. Where fears about coping are a problem then anything new, any demand or task or meeting, becomes a threat-proving situation, too far forward in the mind and affecting rest, relaxation and sleep.

Case Note

A child of eight was seen recently with an acute sleep problem. The family had returned home from an outing and discovered a break-in had occurred. The child's room had been rummaged, along with the rest of the house. Since that time the girl, a sensitive, bright and verbal child, advanced both physically and mentally for her years, had not slept as normally. In the evenings she demanded story after story, was acutely phobic, demanding in the extreme, would not play on her own any more, was only confident when other children were with her and, when eventually off to sleep, would waken at the slightest noise to come into the parents' bed for comfort and security.

In a similar way a child that has been assaulted, caned at school, interfered with or in any way made to feel vulnerable, can in certain sensitive-vulnerable temperaments be quite unable to sleep for long periods of weeks or months. Sometimes parents import fears into a growing child for neurotic reasons and this can create various problems and psychological complications according to the individual.

For some temperaments anything new can be a threat and a problem, especially where bridges are consistently crossed long before troubles occur so that problems are courted or anticipated before they ever become a reality. Adult grief is another common factor in insomnia with loneliness, insecurity, nervousness and a return to an infantile state of vulnerability with the need of a night-light or refusal to sleep alone in the house occurring as a temporary but very real and difficult phase of the grief and sense of loss.

Others are tense before a speech, an interview, a sermon, a wedding, a court-case or an examination and sometimes prior to a flight or a holiday. The arrangements, the preparations, the thinking about it all, the getting ready and the discussions cause tension and insomnia for weeks before the event and sometimes well after it has been completed.

An alert mind, over-involved, too concerned and identified with other people, their problems, worries and demands can always release far too much energy late in the evenings so that surface energy and surface thoughts predominate and cause restless misery during the night hours with chronic insomnia often the outcome.

Anguish

The third major and most misunderstood cause of insomnia is usually confused with the psychological cause and wrongly assumed by both doctor and patient alike to be identical with it. The level of anguish is at the deepest level of man, namely malaise or dis-ease within the inspirational-existential level of being. Sometimes the level is called the spiritual level, but this nomenclature is unsatisfactory because of so much misunderstanding and confusion as to the meaning of the term and therefore it is best avoided. The level exists in everyone and is ubiquitous, one to be integrated and come to terms with, whatever the age or level of awareness.

The problem is one of Life's existence, of mortality, or ageing, of being and not-being, of death as well as the purpose and meaning of life and our way or role in life. When insomnia takes root at this level, it can be the most difficult of all to deal with. It is often closely linked with faith, religion and belief, or the loss of an overall philosophy of life and living. There is almost always dissatisfaction with the material, with things, and often with what has been achieved so far and what has been expressed. There may be profound awareness of self, or doubt, or fear, loneliness and uncertainty – a poignant sense of vulnerability.

There is both the need of people yet a wanting to be alone. Especially there is an almost urgent need of a meaningful dialogue and talk and expression. A need to be, to relate, to exist, to care and to love fully and with meaning and purpose. With existential malaise, as opposed to existential awareness, there may be a sense of restlessness, even when alone, a sense of searching activity, never fully still or able to relax properly with an absence of any inner sanctuary or stillness and sense of peace. In some way the existential malaise causes a sense of seeking for some indefinable other – like a bird without a nest, an eagle without a crag, or even a ball without a socket, reflecting an incompleteness.

There is one situation which makes for peace at this level and this temporary freedom comes from losing the self by becoming totally absorbed in some other activity. This total absorption can be from a book, a play, a film or a relationship. It is never curable but after such a sense of absorption very commonly a good night's sleep follows.

Such a deep level of disturbance gives rise to a variety of apparent outer symptoms and problems such as fear, vertigo, migraine, anxiety, sweating or attacks of collapse and weakness and insomnia. The symptoms always seem psychological but in reality they are not. They are too short-lived, not sufficiently intractable to come within the sphere of true anxiety or neurosis.

Usually such psychological symptoms-apparent are of quite secondary importance and the outcome of an extraordinary sense of vulnerability and sensitivity. Relationships are not interfered with at all, nor is the work area undermined. There is no marriage crisis, the widowed situation has been adjusted to many years before. Sexuality is not impaired, the relationship with friends and interests in general are largely undisturbed. Typical of this level of insomnia is the sudden waking, often in the middle of the night or sometimes from an afternoon nap, in the best of possible situations, feeling wide awake, sweating, panicky or often fearful and vulnerable – and nothing has occurred or is happening to bring about or precipitate the 'attacks' or wakefulness.

Usually they are treated with a variety of tranquillizers which does little to help, causes a greater sense of dependency and vulnerability and often there is worsening of the problem and additional anxiety from the treatment because it is directed at the wrong level and area of malaise.

Homoeopathic Remedies

Lycopodium – For any form of insomnia associated with over-activity of the mind and thought processes and severe anticipatory anxiety.
Chamomilla – Insomnia associated with neuralgic pains in any part of the body, but especially of the face, mouth and gum area with irritability.
Gelsemium – Where there is restless, aching pains, paralysing weakness and a vague sense of panic and anxiety, not necessarily associated with the event.
Ignatia – Whenever grief and loss are contributing factors and anxiety in any form, particularly hysterical in type, is relevant.
Cocculus – There is associated nausea, dizziness or vertigo with an inability to stop chattering or thinking, the mind overactive.
China – Whenever there has been a complete emptying of the energy batteries, depleting relaxa-

tion, and inability to sleep in spite of the need of it. There may have been excessive and prolonged periods of support and caring for others which preceded the problem.

Arsenicum – Chilly exhaustion is the problem with restless waking and fussy concern with trivial matters. Often suddenly awake just after midnight.

Kali Carb. – Here the person wakes up much later between 3 and 5 a.m., depressed, exhausted, lonely or home-sick and worrying themselves into a panic.

Pulsatilla – The time of waking may be before midnight or after, usually very hot although just as easily chilled, restless, weepy and changeable but better for a drink and a biscuit when awake. The arms are often above the head in sleep.

Silicea – Weakness, sweating, often drenching and offensive, palpitations with anxiety, a sense of collapse and devoid of all energy and reserve.

Coffea – Unable to get off to sleep, tense, restless and strung-out, often from too much tea or coffee during the day.

Thuja – For the more odd and bizarre, inexplicable insomnia, sometimes dating since vaccination with stabbing localized pains and a great sense of vulnerability as if the whole body was made of glass.

Lachesis – The sleep is troubled, the person too hot, almost mauve-red in the face, with nightmares of snakes, exhausted, restless, unable to sleep and on waking there is a sense of exhaustion and being aggravated rather than rested.

Lac deflor. – Insomnia when associated with milk allergy in any form.

Opium – Sleepy exhaustion with snoring, constipation and falling asleep at any time of day yet restless and unable to sleep and wind-down at night.

Plumbum – Colicky pains, pins and needles, calf-cramps at night, neuritis or neuralgic pains, constipation and overactivity of the thought processes.

14

Homoeopathy and Emotional Illness (I)

In reality there is no such thing (emotional illness) – only people under pressure with over-stretched emotional pathways causing symptoms of reaction as pressures increase and demands intensify. Typical situations are where there is a threat of some kind – a situation to 'do' something, or 'be' something at the same time conflicting with drives to stay still as before. Non-achievement is the constant threat and with it fear of failure or inability to respond; to be natural when faced with challenges. All change is really life's unfolding and evolution and when there is refusal to accept and to come to terms with it, this must inevitably cause new problems because reality of some kind to some degree has been delayed or denied or put off, causing guilt and often fear, as distorted versions come increasingly to the fore and pressures, instead of being diminished are actually increased by the phantasies that associate and are 'free' to fill the gap of the excluded reality situation.

Deviations, blockages and overspill are inseparable from the whole emotional scene now enacted and put into motion, and are where the problem really starts as a direct counter-reaction to suppression of psychological energy. Other channels are obliged to fill the gap and funnel-off displaced feelings and become alternative conduits for nervous impulse energy flow, although not designed or developed to provide less direct and painful exits for what seems an intolerable, unprepared for, unwelcome, unfamiliar threat and challenge.

Where the direct paths of psychological expression and outlet, response and drive become blocked then too, feelings at all and every level may be unexpressed. Where this becomes a long term chronic attitude it can lead to the most disastrous and, sometimes incurable, illness of every type and pattern.

Case Examples

A woman of 40 – her son was sent to the Falklands and her father became critically ill at the same time – suddenly acutely lost weight and went into a severe and dangerous diabetic crisis (with no previous history of the disease), having suppressed all outward feelings to both emotional situations.

A woman of 28, when her husband of 30 had a coronary, suppressed all outward emotion and reactions and shortly afterwards developed multiple sclerosis.

Pressures build up, of an emotional affective type, needing and demanding immediate release and expression for relief and health, as well as reassurance and feed-back – and these trickle away constantly and chronically through the physical 'other' effluents to irritate and lessen their functioning and efficiency – as with nervous tachycardia, breath-holding attacks, asthma, duodenal ulceration, heart attacks, pain, spasm of every type, weakness, collapse and fainting.

Alternative Pathways

The alternative pathways are chosen for a variety of reasons – not always clear, sometimes from familiar patterns, or because a previous physical illness has so weakened them – that they are more vulnerable and susceptible – for the emotional cuckoo to be deposited within them, gaining entry and then overwhelming normal function or dominating it. Once displaced and re-channelled in this way it is not easy for the body to redirect them back to their normal direct pathways of outlet and expression.

Examples are the bladder in chronic nervous frequency or before an examination; the bowel in nervous diarrhoea, before a new social situation, a first party for the sensitive child; the bronchial tubes in asthma, when there is an emotional demand or threat of some sort; the cardiac impulse pathways in palpitations when there is chronic stress or an anticipated threat situation; the stomach and duodenum in nervous indigestion, where there is underlying tension often of a chronic type and the inability to express it (particularly in anger and rage); the pharynx where there is a nervous lump in the throat and every emotional situation in life is denied and swallowed up at a cost to the individual's comfort and ease.

At the same time, homoeopathic remedies have a uniquely dual action on both these areas of function – the physical pathways – here in emotional illness, stretched to the limit with an emotional charge that is 'foreign' as well as having an intensity that is not part of their usual functioning. The psychological pathway of action of the homoeopathic remedy is well known and the resultant anxiety felt is often because they are blocked and not directly functioning, spilling over into the physical alternatives, changing their usual functioning, to one of physical disarray which is calculated to be unrecognizable from the original pressure-demand situation – but at the same time causing additional different problems – as already described *instead* of fear, anxiety and tension of a psychological type.

Typical examples of the dual action of certain homoeopathic remedies are:

Lycopodium   with action upon the physical bladder as in nervous frequency, as well as such emotional areas as insecurity, anticipatory fear, stage or examination fright, or being the least bit competitive. Hypochondriasis and general overawareness of the self and over-sensitivity is marked.

Natrum Mur   acts upon the larynx as in nervous hoarseness or hysterical loss of the voice, paralysis of one laryngeal chord from nervous reasons – but also associated with depression, tearfulness, anxiety, insecurity, never able to relax or be natural or themselves in any situation in life.

Spigelia   acts upon the heart and circulation, and associated nervous palpitations, but also has activity and resonance with states of sadness, timidity and inability to concentrate.

Nux vomica   is strongly associated with spasm and irritability of the stomach and duodenal lining and with hiatus hernia, heart-burn and spasm as well as the most intense feelings of anger, irritation and short-fuse emotional outbursts.

Pulsatilla is associated with fluid retention and balance, digestion and vasomotor control, and it is also strongly linked with emotional states of passivity, variability, tearfulness and shyness – in public – although sometimes aggression in private.

Homoeopathy uniquely balances both these areas with the single remedy having a predisposition, a resonance and dynamic affinity with the associated emotional states as well as the physical routes and exits taken. It acts as a balancing agent and catalyst to the realignment and outward expression of emotions and feelings, whether suppressed and blocked or inappropriately filtered-off into the physical pathway.

Where symptoms have become 'physical' by over-taxing and over-stretching the physiological pathways by the intrusion of 'foreign' emotional overspill, there is an excess of energy breaking through into the physical, disturbing intrinsic physiological balance and well-being, creating recognizable but physiological expressions of tension and imbalance with symptoms from both – for example, extra-systoles or heart-beats, a racing pulse, sudden fibrillation or flickering of muscle groups in the eye or arm – as there is irritation to normal functioning and at the same time the body attempts to right the imbalance and return to a situation of correction and homoeostasis, to an internal milieu in physiological harmony of functioning.

On the Causes of Emotional Illness

The three major factors are:

(1) Suppression – not always such a problem but the reactions and emotional responses to it can be important.
(2) Negative certainty – with conviction and belief almost certainly ante-dating the acute trigger-precipitating situation by months or even years.
(3) Negative self-imagery – also a much earlier trait and also ante-dating the 'event' by months or years.

Overspill

Note that the simple emotional suppression of a feeling response with displacement into the physical channels and expressions does not in itself create either emotional illness or disease. It does produce a physical expression of a psychological problem or theme, and a psychosomatic condition with the physical pathway conveying the emotional current and psychological energy thread.

For actual emotional illness to occur, further steps are necessary which are different and additional to the provision of an alternative outlet. There must be a disturbed basic relationship with the self which becomes associated and connected with the repression, suppression and denial and other outlets. This disturbance occurs with a disturbed relationship with others, that of being, or relating, and of developing emotionally – of maturing, giving out to others – really of loving so that they become significantly lessened or blocked and denied. Often there is guilt at just being, feeling

88

and expressing, which anger and rage turns inwardly. This is primarily an essential problem for the individual and one which blocks every level of acceptance of self, of being and of existing with any degree of ease and spontaneity. The inner psychological attitudes quite simply is one of 'wait and see', of 'no' or 'can't'. Both they and everything is pre-judged, found wanting and condemned. As a patient told me yesterday who had a breakdown 6 years ago – 'I want to break out and be separate and be a person – not so dominated by my mother, my boss and my boy-friend'. Yet for her, break-out and expressing is inseparable from break-down and illness, because of the intensity of feelings, and terrifies her.

The Causation of Overspill

The English disease of the time of Sir William Osler at the turn of the century was Emphysema and Bronchitis – but it might better have been called 'stiff upper lip' or 'not in front of the children'. The commonest causes of overspill are emotional expressions which are suppressed as soon as there is any level of intensity of emotional situation, either from an 'outside' trigger such as work, family, marriage or achievement, pressure, or an 'inside' one with an anticipated event, meeting, confrontation, expression of an idea, opinion, communication, promotion, fear of failure or not coming up to scratch to anything new, different, challenging.

Grief, shock, fear, assault or trauma (especially psychological, but also physical) may cause a surge of too much feeling, depending upon individual temperament, attitude and maturity, with the threat of being overwhelmed, paralysed, taken over by emotions. There is demand and pressure to control and 'keep in', conflicting strongly with demands to let go, show feelings, even violent ones – just this once – perhaps just this once in a lifetime – to show the others.

The physical alternatives, by their irritation and anger within, often give expression to angry looking, irritable, physical expressions at a whole variety of levels. There may be a red and angry looking skin eruption or anal irritation, needing clawing at with finger nails to get some relief; the eruption expressing the psychological conflict as well as providing a temporary and often doubtful, solution to an acute emotional problem, also provokes different and greater worries and problems, making demands on the object of the psychological feelings commonly, so that they too feel paralysed, worried or guilty and responsible. Eventually there may be no solution to the underlying psychological feelings, as the same problem keeps on emerging inevitably and differently, but wearing a different hat or metaphor on each occasion.

Negative Certainty

As mentioned, this always pre-dates the acute emotional outburst, usually an internal one. There has usually been conviction at a whole variety of levels, which is self-critical relating to self-expression, physical appearance, individuality, ability and everything that is at all spontaneous and unique within the self. The case is pre-judged and found erring so to speak, unacceptable and wanting, beyond argument, question or doubt; sapping confidence, sense of being, feeling acceptable and lovable, which empties relationships and ease in any aspect of the personal being.

Examples of Negative Certainty

(1) An agoraphobic patient is totally convinced that she will faint, collapse, fall down or die if she is more than about one mile from her home, especially if held up by traffic or a short queue when she feels worse – intensely irritated, impatient and overwhelmed by emotion.

(2) A schizophrenic man is convinced that his feelings and thoughts can be read by others and that this feeling is no part of his illness or delusions – "it is a fact, and was told to him once by a priest and was written in the Bible. Some people can definitely do this!" The obscene homosexual thoughts he has are in a similar way 'put' there by others and make him shy and self-conscious because he is really attracted to women and not to boys or other men.

Negative Self-Imagery

This is a serious and usually long-standing disorder of self-perception which, when severe, can lead to severe problems such as anorexia, schizophrenia or depression, with lack of confidence and withdrawal. There is a separation of actual self from phantasy-image, usually a distorted one which is not corrected at a reality level, so that confusion occurs and individuality becomes quite unacceptable. It is always based on phantasy-imagery, causing the distortion of self with infantile, magical-omnipotent thinking so that self-assessment is incorrect, undermined and an easy relaxed attitude

91

impossible. When severe, it leads to the most enormous self-consciousness, shyness and problems of space between self and others, ease of being, expressing, and a sense of negative criticism from others, and self-dislike. When severe, as in psychotic or puerperal conditions, there can be a delusional accompaniment and association about the body; its size, shape, smell and boundaries.

Examples of Negative Self-Imagery

(1)   A patient had a long-term negative sado-masochistic relationship with her talented but psychotic partner. She was unable to break away from him and leave, although he told her that she was ugly, dressed badly, and would soon lose her job. She could not leave because she was so unsure of herself from negative self-imagery that she partly believed him, because he said what she thought about herself and confirmed it externally. She became depressed, lost confidence further and was eventually psychologically paralysed – unable to look at herself, her partner and her own negatives.

(2)   An anorexic girl was so convinced at 17 that she was fat, overweight and ugly, she started to diet although at the time she was only 8 stones. Her periods stopped, her thighs sunk in and one eye became displaced and shrunken from loss of orbital fat. Now, 2 years later, her weight is 9 stones, she has no desire to fast but has periods of excessive eating followed by crash diets, but it is less severe. The periods have not returned nor the thigh fat or that of the orbit, and there is danger of permanent disfigurement.

(3)   A hypochondriacal over-sensitive youth was so convinced that he will fail his exams that he

made no real effort to work or to try and cover the syllabus. He does not work throughout the year or revise comprehensibly, relying on a few 'spot' questions learned parrot-fashion at the last minute, having given up trying because of conviction of failure and negative self-imagery.

(4) A stockbroker is so nervous before a public speech that he is paralysed with fear and anxiety for weeks beforehand, yet he is highly successful and able – chairman of his own company, highly competent and knowledgeable. The speech is to be on his own subject and one that he has arranged to stimulate business and to put over his image to potential clients. But, at 50, he is still dominated by early infantile fears and by a weak, fearful, timid self-imagery, so that he also leaves the speech until the last moment, creating additional pressures. The familiar 'devil you know' here, anxiety, tension, dread, negatives about the self-image – in this case are not better than the one you don't know – the new, unknown situation of the speech and questions afterwards, and it is a costly price that is paid in terms of comfort and ease, and sometimes in terms of loss of business and revenue if the actual performance is also undermined. In general, it is not the event that is so painful but the anticipatory period leading up to it where the negatives can dominate in a familiar yet highly damaging and limiting negative way.

15

Homoeopathy and Emotional Illness (II)

Dreams and the Patient

Freud called the dream 'the royal road to the unconscious'. Here are some recent examples from patients, taken before an acute crisis in their differing illnesses which illustrate to some degree the relationship of the dream to both the physical state as well as the mental – which is the major unique property of the homoeopathic potency as well, so that both dream and remedy have a duality about their functioning and expression, and therefore a direct relationship which is often used in prescribing the choice of remedy.

I A Patient with Multiple Sclerosis

The patient was on the beach walking with wife and child. Suddenly an enormous tidal wave came in without warning, sweeping away the family, and my patient only surviving by clinging desperately onto some iron-railings. The very next morning both legs collapsed; there was loss of sensation and movement, and he was unable to walk again for several months before there was some recovery.

The legs were cold, damp, clammy and sweating, feeling full of fluid, soggy and as if water-logged, although there was not true oedema or swelling. The body seemed to be retaining fluid and was distended within the tissues of the face and under both eyes – the patient was as if drowned within his own tissue fluid. It is interesting to recall here that any major disturbance of sodium-ion balance within the body also acts reciprocally upon the key potassium ions, which are indispensable for electrical discharge at the neuromuscular end-plates, and essential for strength of muscular functioning. When the sodium ion levels are high, potassium is low and vice versa, and low potassium means paralysis of muscular functioning and weakness.

The dream shows a massive influx of sodium ions totally overwhelming the body and isolating the patient from the family – representing his integration and other balancing units as part of his totality or family. Massive tidal inflow of sodium meant potassium ions depleted to nil, with total muscular inertia and paralysis – the tissues drowned in their own accumulated fluid in an attempt to wash out the excessive sodium, as is often the case with the excessive thirst of the salt addict – in an attempt to dilute and excrete the sodium ion excesses. The major remedy from the homoeopathic repertory which links with the dream and clinical picture is potentized sea or ocean and salt – namely, *Natrum mur*.

Second Dream

That night the patient had a second dream which linked with the first – he dreamed that he was an

Indian beggar, both legs amputated and having to propel himself on a rubber tyre with his hands, his palms protected by a kind of metal hand plate to prevent excessive damage as he pushed himself around.

The significance of the metal iron comes into both dreams and is surely not without significance – the iron railing of the first dream – which he clings to, and the hand-protective plates of the second. There is a life-saving protective quality about the metal, and it may be that what he needed to balance the overwhelming sodium influx and tissue paralysis and drowning, was the metal Iron or perhaps Lead or *Zincum* in homoeopathic potency.

II   A Patient with Motor Neurone Disease

The night before a severe exacerbation and paralytic episode of both throat and tongue so that dribbling was pronounced and swallowing difficult – the speech even more slurred and drunken-sounding – the following dream occurred.

He was back at sea again as a naval commander in the war, and was giving orders to torpedo a nearby naval destroyer. But the vessel he was ordering to be sunk was one of his own fleet and on his side. Here was a chilling warning dream and forecast of what was shortly to follow, or was it indeed already being prepared within the depths of the physiological and psychological self? There was an attack – ultimately on an extension of the self – rather than on an enemy or another. There was a massive piece of physiological masochism with a devastating weapon – again played out on the ocean which might indicate *Natrum mur* or a

Natrum salt for the remedy, and at the same time with metal used for the attacking device – rather than any helpful salvation for health or positive ally.

After the dream, the whole illness entered into a final and terminal downhill pattern so that irreversible paralysis and a negative incurable course occurred. The dream was part of the patient's totality, and illustrates possible remedies for consideration to be taken into account with the other psychological and physical totality as part of the prescribing picture, the dream illustrating the dynamics and its symbols, the sinking of the self-ship and how health and all progress was finally being sunk and torpedoed.

III   A Patient with a Mild Congenital Spastic Condition

Here, the main symptoms of the patient (aged 26) were slight muscular weakness in the left leg, lack of co-ordination in the left hand and inability to fully concentrate for long on any task in hand or to follow instructions through coherently and definitely.

In the dream she was engaged to her boy-friend and he was driving back from his job to be with her. Half way to her he was involved in a crash, was killed, and did not get through to her, of course. This was a very repetitive pattern of her dreams – someone or something was lost or killed or blocked from getting through to her.

Here is a likely explanation of the dream's symbolism, apart from the obvious wish-fulfilment and fear of loss regarding the boy-friend was also an expression of underlying neuro-muscular impulse processes, of the message from the brain that does not get through properly or only partially; is blocked or interfered with as part of the spastic condition, due in fact, to a very rapid and precipitate birth, accounting for the inco-ordination and weakness (the 'fiancé' neuromuscular impulse and signal) because the partner, or the one proposed to complete the totality of stimulus-response, did not arrive because it had a crash or accident.

The Physical Exits used by Suppressed Emotional Energies

Each of the following physical exits can also be related to a homoeopathic remedy which has resonance or vital reaction with it along part or whole of its tract from the physiological properties of the mother substance of origin, retaining these qualities of site of stimulation whatever the dilution or potency. The homoeopathic remedy is also related to a whole series of emotional states of psychological energy and expression, and where the physical exit chosen and emotional state match, then there is a high degree of consistency, and the probability that the individual and the remedy match with the particular remedy indicated either at once, or at some time in the future.

Some Common Examples with Indicated Remedies, with Associated Pathways having a High Level of Emotional Activity

1. **The Gastro-Intestinal Tract** – Typical symptoms include indigestion, flatulence, heartburn, peptic ulcer, spasm, acidity, wind, pain, loss of

appetite, nervous vomiting, nausea, nervous diarrhoea, nervous incontinence.

Arg. Nit., Arsenicum, Nux vom., Kali carb.

2. **Genito-Urinary Pathway** – Typical symptoms include impotence, frigidity, nervous frequency, pruritis.

Lycopodium, Natrum mur., Sepia, Berberis.

3. **The Laryngo-Pharyngeal Tract** – Typical symptoms include nervous cough, nervous laryngitis, nervous hoarseness, sense of lump in the throat, dryness in the throat, inability to swallow.

Natrum mur., Causticum, Kali bic.

4. **The Hormonal Routes** – Typically diabetes, thyrotoxicosis, dysmenorrhoea.

Natrum mur., Sepia, Pulsatilla.

5. **The Pulmonary Tract** – Typical symptoms include asthma, hay-fever, nervous cough or tickle, shortness of breath when tense.

Bryonia, Phosphorus, Lycopodium, Arsenicum.

6. **The Cardio-Circulatory Tract** – Typical symptoms include palpitations, tachy-cardia, angina with emotion.

Aurum met., Spigelia.

7. **Vaso-Motor Tracts** – Blushing, sweating, hot-flushes, fainting.

Silicea, Pulsatilla.

8. **The Muscular-Skeletal System** – Typical symptoms include pain, spasm, cramp, low back pain, tics, nervous paralysis.

Calcarea, Nux vom., Cuprum, Zincum met.

9. **The Joints** – Frozen shoulder, rheumatoid arthritis.

Rhus tox.

10. **The Skin** – Nervous eczema, urticaria, nervous rashes.

Sulphur, Belladonna.

In conclusion, the homoeopathic approach to illness is that, however tangible the externals, the physicals, to some degree every problem has a spark of the intangible, the indefinable, the psychological, and mentals within it – for nothing is purely and totally physical – the psychological thread is always there as a contributory thread however minor or major to give a lead to timing and action of the problem.

Similarly, every intangible problem, however obviously psychological, contains within it the germ of a physical element which responds to the intangibles – because they are inseparable really – the bowel or stomach in a nervous or anticipatory state, the skin perhaps in a psychotic problem. The link with the homoeopathic remedy is that each remedy, however tangible the potency, however low the dilution and detectable the mother-substance, nevertheless, at such low dilutions, has a link and a resonance with the psychological even if not very marked or obvious.

Similarly, in the highest intangible potencies of the CM or MM range of infinites, there are always significant physical tangible actions, properties and links. It is this duality of the homoeopathic potencies that makes them so unique and relevant to the illnesses of modern man, and is also why they are so very effective.

16

Homoeopathy and Psychiatry

Man is inseparable from all that is *homo sapiens* – intelligence, sensitivity and awareness. Inevitably and for all of us, such feelings sometimes include grief, pain, loss, fear and destructive impulses. Homoeopathy is a total, truly holistic therapy, an approach to the person as an individual, as an entirety, not as a collection of fragments, 'bits and pieces' in isolation. When a problem seems uncomplicated and straightforward, a graze, fall, cut or sprain, nevertheless there are always some degree of associated feelings and emotions present. These may be quite superficial, on the surface and fleeting, understandable reactions to a shock situation. But underlying, deeper psychological attitudes and motivations can also be involved and throw light on other, similar incidents, which do not fall quite into the category of accident-proneness. These are the expression of underlying anxieties and tensions, often unconscious, perhaps a flight from feeling able to confidently deal with a particular relationship, or a new situation. The physical may seem more acceptable than the emotional when there appears to be an insurmountable difficulty or obstacle, which cannot be confronted or dealt with because of fear, lack of maturity, support, courage or confidence. In such cases it is questionable whether much will be gained for the patient by simply treating locally, a graze with *Calendular*, *Bellis* for a sprain or using *Arnica* for shock. Homoeopathic help is needed for the underlying reasons and causes, the lack of confidence and fear, perhaps a difficulty in being open with feelings and vulnerability within the family. Diagnosis is always the key, and diagnosis in depth as well as breadth is what homoeopathy is concerned with. Once the diagnosis is right, with attention to detail and individuality, then the right remedy can be more easily and confidently prescribed for a total diagnosis and a total therapy.

All of this brings into focus the frequent dilemma of the homoeopath and the problem of just what should be prescribed for the problem and at what potency. A common condition such as ankle sprain, with associated reactions of shock, fear and tension needs careful thought. Should *Arnica* or *Aconitum* be given for the immediates, the local tendon reactions, the fear, shock and pain, or should *Ruta* be given for the tendon over-extension, perhaps *Calcarea* when the problem is known to be recurrent, or should it be *Kali Carb* with its known affinity for accident-proneness, particularly in left-sided problems. *Nux vomica* might also be considered when the predominant symptoms are spasm and tension with tears of irritability and where a 'pique' of anger preceded the event and injury.

The common difficulty that all prescribers meet in such cases is should the treatment be purely local? *Apis* for swelling, *Rhus Tox* for stiffness, better for warmth and movement, or should it be a treatment, perhaps the patient's constitutional which incorporates the patient's temperament and personality as well as physical areas of vulnerability and the Achilles heel of the patient in times of stress and pressure?

This is the problem and often the difficulty for the prescriber. There may be no easy answer for doctor or patient alike and the answer undoubtedly rests on sound diagnosis, experience and clinical judgement in the final analysis.

You may ask at this point – well how do we decide the right remedy?, and having decided the treatment, at what potency, and does it matter if the remedy is an exact fit? or what constitutes the right remedy and should the psychologicals be considered in *every* case? and if so to what degree?

None of these are easy questions and the answers are not always immediately obvious. In general though, double-check your prescription for an obvious physical and local condition by making sure that there is a good match with the mentals of the patient and conversely when treating an obvious psychological state, make quite sure that the prescription also fits the physicals and modalities as well as the mentals. In this way you will be in the best and most balanced position for an overall assessment of the patient as a totality and not prescribing on a part or a portion of the whole.

In general the psychologicals ought at least to be considered and thought about in every case, especially where the emotions, or mentals, as Hahnemann called them, as a result of his early psychiatric experience, obviously play a role in bringing the patient to the doctor, the adult into crisis, the child running to the mother.

The danger of ignoring the emotional factor is that the results of prescribing will be mediocre or unsatisfactory, that a 'nuts and bolts' homoeopathy will ensue based on the part and the superficial, resembling a suppressive, allopathic approach, rather than a holistic one. Failure to consider any problem in sufficient depth, reduces the potential of the remedies to put the patient back into equilibrium.

Homoeopathy is a natural, biological stimulus to health because it is in resonance with man's essential nature and make-up, the physical as well as the psychological and because it uses subtle, non-tangible energies, it is also in resonance with the inspirational-creative, indefinable aspects. Its actions do not put health or physiological functioning at risk because it supports all natural functioning with a gentle stimulus to tonicity and flow, rather than being inhibiting and alien to it. The apparent aggravation of a healing crisis is a result of release of flow, rather than the outcome of a disharmonious condition, and in that sense an aggravation is an intense, but harmonious stimulus to a return to natural rhythms.

Homoeopathy is the only natural therapy which fully mobilizes the psychological as well as the energy flows of the physical and this is quite specific for every remedy and the reason why the repertory begins with the deeper mentals and then the physicals.

Every homoeopathic remedy, by definition contains mental and physical resonance because there is no condition in man that is 100% physical or entirely, 100% psychological. Each contains some element of the other and the remedies reflect this complexity of man. Every homoeopathic potency has duality of action to match the inter-play of physical depths with the vicissitudes, depths and layers of individuality and the infinite variety of alternating thoughts, feelings, actions and motivations.

Any of the psychological areas may become 'fixed' and emerge as physical disfunction as much as a psychological condition. As an emotional disturbance often reflects a physical imbalance, a physical change also reflects the individual, his or her life-style, their situation, past and degree of overall balance and health. Such changes reflect the individual, temperament, genetic make-up and maturity and homoeopathy has the capacity to act positively within all these inter-relating layers to free stasis or blockage within them.

Some of the best known remedies which are daily prescribed for psychological problems include the following.

Lycopodium, which acts strongly on anticipatory, futuristic anxieties and fears about a tomorrow which paralyses today. Physically it acts on the lung functioning, the intestinal organs of digestion, with a particular preference for right-sided areas of the body indicating its specificity of action on the left cerebral hemisphere.

Natrum mur acts on fears for today, for any involvement, closeness, on being natural and spontaneous, the expression in the now of the authentic self and any weakened sense of personal identity and vulnerability preventing relaxation, ease and freedom from tension. Its physical action is on the heart and circulation, the fluid balance, kidneys, skin, joints and on every organ of the body to some degree.

Aurum met. has action on the past, on past guilt, past regrets and past feelings of failure which over-shadow the drive for life, love and going on. It also has very strong action on the heart and articulations.

Nux vomica affects both the past and the future within its sphere of mentals with an intensity, leading to spasm. Irritability and guilt as well as short-fuse precipitate actions with inability to ever delegate are well-known psychological limitations which make for many of the physical disabilities as well as the emotional problems which occur with others. Its action is in many ways similar in the physical sphere with withholding leading to tension, tightness and a reluctance to let go. Tension headaches, lumbago and constipation are just some of the common manifestations of the temperament and the specificity of the remedy's action.

Psychological illness is simply the reaction of over-activity and over-stimulation in a particular area of the mentals. In this way there is disturbed balance because of an outpouring of feelings into one area which has to compensate by the formation of warning symptoms in order to survive the tidal flow of emotions, usually inappropriate and excessive. The individual understandably feels in a position of imbalance; one of anguish and tension with fear, restlessness, even delusion as perception and judgement gets caught up in a flood of feeling which distorts, weakens and overwhelms the emotional layers and their usual state of balance.

The reasons are complex and may be either physical or psychological in origin. All the skills of the physician are needed to diagnose the true roots

107

and origins of a disturbed psychological state. This is important in homoeopathy because traditionally the homoeopath has always tried to go back to the beginnings of every problem under treatment – physical or mental. In a psychological state it is not only important, but essential to try and do this because a remedy that matches the initial trauma, also acts upon the initial earliest knots of the disturbance and once these are loosened, more of the patient is available and accessible to support the overall processes of cure.

When the causes are physical, as after an acute traffic trauma, industrial accident, a fracture, infection, toxic or parasitic state, or drug-induced, leading to an acute allergic reaction, then homoeopathy may be less effective. A physical treatment may be more indicated, as plastic surgery, replacement of fluids and electrolyte correction, perhaps surgery or an orthopaedic intervention. But this is not always the case and sometimes homoeopathy may be the treatment of choice, for example in an acute psychological state, the outcome of influenza, glandular fever or mumps, when the specific nosode in homoeopathic potency can bring about a rapid cure. In very acute mental states, urgent treatment is needed because of the confusion, fear, delusional aspects and homoeopathy is less effective when under pressure. In such cases hospitalization may be the only answer, sometimes with sedation or restraint.

But there are homoeopathic remedies for acute mental states which are very valuable and can put the most disturbed patient back into balance provided that it is given early enough, in time to take effect and in the correct potency and naturally that it matches the overall symptom profile of the patient. Some of the commonest examples include *Belladonna*, *Stramonium*, *Hyoscyamus*, the triad of *Nash*. But there are others too such as *Aconitum*, *Cantharis*, *Tarantular hisp.* and each needs to be carefully differentiated to be effective.

Sometimes the prescribing rests only on the odd, rare and peculiar symptom to give accuracy of prescribing. For example the sense of a nail being driven slowly through the skull, causing the most intense and constant localized pain, or that the body is made of glass which is fragmenting inside, indicates *Thuja*. Without specificity of prescribing there is inaccuracy, results are mediocre and disappointing.

The Advantages of Homoeopathy for the Patient with a Psychological Problem

1. It speeds up and facilitates the processes of cure and insight, gaining valuable time for both patient and doctor.
2. Homoeopathy facilitates and supports the processes of internal balance and integration, both physiologically and psychologically. It can release rigid or blocked static states where there is a long term problem.
3. Psychologically, homoeopathy supports the processes of insight, because it acts to stimulate a healthier re-formation and re-structuralization of psychological processes and patterns into new, more flexible, associations which reduce rigid, negative unhealthy attitudes. It stimulates new perceptions, which are more reality-based and not the outgrowth of a disturbed or withdrawn psychological state.

4. In many ways homoeopathy also arrests the processes which make for a more interminable course or a problem of chronicity because it limits rigid attitudes. *Natrum mur* in the correct potency is of particular value in this respect.
5. Because homoeopathy helps prevent chronicity, it supports positive changes or shifts within the patient's conceptualization and understanding, so that change or movement does not immediately revert back to an unhealthy pattern after a brief period of improvement. With homoeopathy the changes that occur tend to be permanent ones, because more out-going, reality-based attitudes and relationships are supported by the remedies.
6. Homoeopathy stimulates flexible attitudes which give greater ease within relationships generally. This reduces spasm and hard attitudes, as long as the right remedy has been prescribed for the patient and sufficiently 'high'.

Time is needed in homoeopathy for adequate consultation time, for the patient to communicate and to emerge, in a sympathetic, non-judgmental setting, that is consistent. This reassures the patient and gives time for new material to become free, available for discussion and thought. The patient also needs time to make changes in attitude that have often taken years to form. Also there must be adequate time allowed between remedies, with a restrained, light, homoeopathic approach that gives the remedies sufficient time for action, only giving a further prescription when there is a clear-cut indication for it.

Consistency implies that the patient sees the same doctor each time, who knows the case and where there is a communicating dialogue and a caring between doctor and patient. Constant changes of doctor during any treatment are counter-productive and like constant changes of remedy, lead to second-class homoeopathy that is a disservice to the whole approach.

In this way phobic conditions, depression, anguish and anxiety can be treated and improved, provided that the approach and remedy are correct for the specific emotional problem. Where the damage is more deep-seated, remote, perhaps from childhood the correct prescription may be the one that goes back to the origins of the problem, treating the initial trauma and imbalance, because at the time, it was not fully resolved, or even acknowledged, because of denial, indifference or ignorance. When the origins are treated as well as the prevailing symptoms, with a remedy that takes into account the physical as well as the mentals, it can resonate with and untie knots from the past, putting the patient back into balance again to find a more authentic identity.

There are no recipes for homoeopathic prescribing in psychological problems. Each formulation depends upon the individual, their predominant symptoms and the preoccupations, reactions and the intensity of mood at the time.

Major Remedies that Often Play a Role and have Strong Mental Resonance

Arnica
For psychological bruising, anguish, pain and exhaustion after a psychological shock or fairly

recent traumatic encounter where the patient feels that they 'came off badly', did not adequately express themselves at the time or cope well. As a result, they feel damaged in terms of their self image and self-esteem to the extent that their psychological expression is stiff, stilted or brittle.

Arsenicum

This plays a frequent role in the treatment of emotional problems and supports *Natrum mur* because it too has a lot of stiffness and rigidity of attitudes. Control is emphasized, of self and others with the emphasis on appearance and order. In general they are much more confident and outgoing, other-seeking than *Natrum*. The temperament is combined with a characteristic overactivity of body and mind with considerable energy availability of a nervous kind which quickly leads to exhaustion. Much of their chilliness and sensitivity to cold, the poor circulation, is due to stress causes as much as physiological reasons.

Pulsatilla

Pulsatilla, like *Natrum*, is valuable where there is retention of attitudes and control, combined with variability. Fluids and the psychological self are both retained which makes for much of the typical *Pulsatilla* vulnerability. Like *Natrum*, they can never really be themselves and must always put on an 'act', a 'show' to appease or please, which is always depleting. The psychological imbalance leads to a sensation of being 'swallowed up' so that claustrophobic feelings, fear of lifts, enclosed spaces, of flying are frequent together with considerable general embarrassment and inappropriate guilt. The typical *Pulsatilla* make-up is one of weakness, vulnerability and over-dependency. There is psychological weakness because parts of the self are not free and available, because of suppression and denial so that only premature or partial involvements occur. This often causes complicated highly emotional triangles which vary in intensity and closeness from one moment to the other.

There are other remedies which also have strong mentals and the following have strong mental resonance with problems of excitement and over-activity.

Lilium tig.
Cannot concentrate or think about matters in hand. Tend to act without thought. Hering describes them as overactive, walking fast as if 'by instinct'. They feel hurried but don't know why. Forgetful, can't make decisions, over-dependent on others. Nearly always irritable.

Rhus tox.
In general they tend to be brisk, hasty, quick and trembling.

Sulphur
Resembles *Rhus* in hastiness and restlessness. The mind is a ragbag of unrealistic ideas and plans, usually disorganized and showing the typical *Sulphur* untidiness and lack of reality. There is an unhealthy idealization of their unreal and disorganized thought flow.

Viol. tric.
Everything is rushed and quick, as if driven by inward fears. Restlessness.

Calcarea

An obsessional, anxious restless is typical with a preoccupation with minute detail to the exclusion of reality at times. Thinking is repetitive and lassitude and exhaustion are present at every level. They are often confident and strong in mind and intention, but this quickly gives way to lack of will and the strength to carry an initiative to its conclusion and outcome.

Opium

Often associated with a lively overactivity and strength with a red face and glistening eye (*Belladonna*). Useful in mania. At other times there is the typical *Opium* drowsiness.

Bovista

Indicated for manic moods, where there is the desire to fight everyone.

Spongia

For irritable overactivity and an irresistible desire to sing in a mood of excessive hilarity. Absent-minded and indisposed to be involved in any kind of work or activity.

Aloes

There is overactivity associated with great general rushing around and activity with excessive cheerfulness.

Laurocerasus

For overactivity and merry high humour. They feel refreshed in mind and body as part of the surge of energy and overactivity of a hypomanic kind.

Platina
Overactivity with haughty indifference, looking down upon others with a cheerful, confident state which alternates with feelings of depression and despair.

Benzoic ac.
For overactivity which is quickly followed by anxiety.

Tarentula hisp.
For extreme forms of overactivity of a hypomanic type with a tearing destructiveness and impulses towards violence.

17

Emotional Problems of Infancy and Childhood

Infantile Anxiety

Anxiety in the child is a psychological situation where the child feels alienated from his or herself so that both identity and security are threatened, leading to panic, tension, turmoil or fear. Most of the anxiety is about being unable to get back to the whole, undivided sense of self and identity, to a feeling of being, 'realness' and existence.

The insecurity which results, leads to malaise and anguish, a sense of being separated from the real self so that confidence is overwhelmed by overpowering waves of feelings, leaving the child thrown off balance and depressed because life lacks direction, shape or meaning.

Because of the insecurity the child tries to manipulate others in a bid to establish love and security through others and this may give a hysterical or more dramatic shape to the anxiety and its manifestations.

Causes

Always a function of innate strength and vital energy, resilience and confidence and external pressure. *Fear*, *fright* or *loss* of essential security which is undermined or never solidly established because of weak, shifting home-life, sibling relationships, or peer-group changes. Hereditary factors as with over-sensitivity and possibly fastidiousness. Home security either absent or weak from a variety of causes and lacks. Physical illness as brain damage, a physical congenital condition with repeated hospitalizations.

Symptoms

The child may be phobic, clinging or obsessional at play or in the arrangement of his or her room or toys with excessive neatness and arrangement. Avoidance and shyness is marked. Sometimes a child hides in cupboards, or under the bed, especially in any new, strange or unexpected situation which is unfamiliar and also insecure. There is dislike of change, fear of strangers, new children or visitors in the house. Friends may be few and associated with rather controlled, stereotyped games aimed at the control of danger or fear. Physical symptoms include migraine, abdominal pain, spasm, insomnia, bed-wetting or a return to soiling. There is often fear of the dark, of school, or being away from home, of a new teacher or of any change, tending to hide away from strangers. Repetitive games are the rule, routine activities and play, rather than anything daring, imaginative or inventive. Fear of school, of classes, of being alone with one particular parent or when apart from the mother – for example when she is talking with a friend or neighbour, gives rise to provocative and often irritating behaviour at the time.

Fastidious and faddy with food, and there is an over-protective attitude to the mother, with fear of her becoming ill, getting hurt or dying. In general, the pattern of behaviour, even when at home and apparently secure, is for a whimpering, restless behaviour, with crying and undue exaggerated shyness with strangers. Truanting, anti-social behaviour, eating coal or dirt, playing with fire and matches are also common. Nightmares are frequent, the child waking or unable to get off to sleep, seeing ghosts, shapes, or danger, restless and crying, coming into the parent's bed, before eventually falling into a light sleep.

Infantile Hypochondriasis

Symptoms
When severe, there may be phobic obsessional features with anxiety breaking through into every aspect of life – physical as with eating, and imaginative with a severely limited creative expression of the self in terms of thought, speech and ideas. Mild cases may experience only minor hypochondriasis, with over-sensitive, 'allergic' reactions to food or new situations. Eczema, diarrhoea, indigestion and Monday morning nervous 'tummy' are all common. In general, even in mild cases, there is some nausea, spasm or pain at the least change of routine.

Suppressed anxiety leads to loose bowel problems which if severe, may become chronic. Suppressed reactions can also evoke an angry eczema skin reaction, rather than a show of rage or feelings. Such blocked feelings can be damaging, limiting to personality growth, healthy maturation and security.

The least physical pain, discomfort or change is a stimulus to anxiety and to fear of illness and sickness. These fears and phobic symptoms control and limit the environment by a process of manipulation as the internal aspects are given external form by a variety of threatening situations. Typical areas are a fear of travelling, school, examinations, the doctor or dentist. Also pets, insects, bridges, flying or heights may also become focus areas.

Recommended Remedies for Anxiety of the Infant and Young Child

Borax (Borate of Sodium)
Agitated nervousness, can't concentrate, especially after lunch. Changeable and restless, moving from one room or thing to another. Mood is also variable – from tears to laughter (*Pulsatilla*). Irritable and especially worse, clutching at the mother when she leans down to put the child to bed. (Note *Gelsemium* clutches the mother all the time.) Worse for noise, easily startles, and for downward movement of any kind whatsoever.

Calcarea (Carbonate of Lime)
Weakness with inability to sustain concentrated effort. Slow, late and delayed in everything – as much psychological maturity as the physical milestones. Cries easily, is over-fearful and anxious. Weakness is marked. Has sudden impulses – to run wildly down the stairs or jump through a window.

In contrast, the child can also spend hours with one meaningless repetitive game or toy – playing at the same movements – will pick up pins for hours. They are generally preoccupied with insignificant detail and are always worse for cold, for intellectual tasks and better for being constipated.

Calc. Phos. (Phosphate of Lime)

Depressive anxiety, emerging as a nervous collapse or weakness. Irritable and miserable, they often appear rather dull or stupid and can't comprehend what is being asked. At the same time they flash-up (*Phosphorus* component) into rage at being thwarted or criticized (cp. *Ignatia*, *Phos. Ac.*). Worse for damp, for thinking about their worries and problems and better for heat or sleep.

Gelsemium (Yellow Jasmine)

Slow, sleepy, disliking effort and movement. The brain feels 'thick' and congested. They can't concentrate and just want to be left alone in peace, undisturbed. Typically they prefer their own company and solitude (*Natrum Mur.*). Lazy and indolent, at times too lazy to think, the presence of anyone else, exhausts them (cp. *Sepia* where others irritate). First day at school fears and examination 'funk'. The nervous child wants to be held all the time, clutching fearfully and tightly.

Infantile Restlessness

Causes

Either unknown, or associated with a quick oversensitive, temperament, closely resembling one of the parents. There may have been a traumatic birth, sometimes a precipitate delivery, with an

120

early rupture of the membranes and loss of fluid, with a prolonged, exhausting labour and the use of instruments. Sometimes there is a history of a fall or concussion in early childhood. In others, restlessness follows an acute infective condition such as mumps, chicken pox, or meningitis.

Symptoms

These are usually of a tireless child, who never wants to rest for long or to sleep in the evenings. Either at home or in the surgery, they sit only for a moment, then move from one object to another, unable to read or play quietly, demanding attention or to touch, pull and explore, which resents parental control or interference. They touch, explore and want to handle everything, one thing after another, but rarely any one thing in depth. At times they can be difficult to handle or control. A mother may often resort to bribery with sweets or the promise of presents to control or passify, but like the threat of punishment, such techniques are only effective, if at all for the brief moments, and often not at all.

Antimonium Tartrate (Tartrate of Antimony and Potash)

There is restless excitement of the patient and sometimes the whole family. The general home atmosphere may be one of busy restless excitement and impatience. There is little time for anything and a quick prescription and fast diagnosis are required. The doctor as much as everyone is under pressure and everything is in a great hurry (*Medorrhinum*) so that thinking and responses must be rapid.

Chamomilla (German Chamomile)

There is an irritable resentful anger and spiteful impatience, with dislike of being interrupted. Intolerance of others in the environment is common, especially when they have something to say. They dislike being interrupted and can be angered to the point of a temper tantrum. Anxious, restless, agitated, over-sensitive and impressionable, they are exasperated by the least contradiction or pain. The young child is naughty, almost beyond tolerance, tryingly capricious, wanting everything it sees and having a tantrum whenever refused or frustrated in the least way. The child tries to cry until it obtains its way and then rejects when given-into. Only quiet when held or carried, they may also respond to walking. There is insomnia with the agitation, and a low tolerance level of pain or frustration. Nash recommends *Arsenicum alb* (chill and weakness), *Rhus tox* (agitation, better for movement) and *Chamomilla* as the major remedies for restless agitation. *Cina* has similar restless irritability to *Chamomilla* but dislikes being carried.

Jalap (Jalap)

The child is quite good during the day but screams or is particularly restless and difficult at night.

Rheum (Rhubarb)

Another useful child remedy, where there is impatience, the child desires everything and cries a great deal. Sour-smelling diarrhoea, vomit and sweat are also characteristic.

Phobias and Hypochondriasis

Causes

Often there has been an acute fear or trauma, perhaps an early loss or separation from a twin or sibling, or an acute illness or hospitalization, evacuation in the wartime, or the loss is more psychological as another child has grown and developed apart or in new areas. Such an illness, separation or 'event', may be used by the child to confirm their own 'badness', rather than to re-affirm more positive thinking. Ambivalent phantasies and sadistic or punishment themes can be stimulated and reinforce fears of attack or retaliation affecting psychological growth and development at its very roots. In many cases, there has been no obvious cause or apparent trauma and no damage can be recalled, but one or both parents is phobic in some area which becomes attached to the child. The phobic limitations of the parent affected may be re-enacted, including their processes of identification and reality understanding.

Argentum Nit. (Nitrate of Silver)

There is a combination of fatigue, irritability and depression. Everything is rushed and done in a hurry (*Med*) and a constant state of fear, especially of not having enough time to complete a particular task in hand. Other remedies in a hurry are *Medorr.*, *Nat. mur.*, *Nux. vom.*, *Sulph.*, *Alumina*, *Mercuriua*, *Ant. tart*. Fear of public appearances and stage fright (*Gelsemium*). Other fears are that the houses will collapse, of madness or being buried alive, the child is in a hurry because dangers are sensed and felt to be menacing. There may be

123

disturbing impulses to throw him or herself from a high building, or being drawn by water. These are impulses however, rather than true suicidal tendencies. There is agoraphobia, and diarrhoea from going into a new situation.

Other remedies with specific fears.

Gelsemium – fear of public places
Aconitum – crowds
Belladonna – dogs
Nux Vom – knives
Baryta Carb – other children
Psorinum – misfortune in general
Gelsemium – examination, stage-fright.

Lycopodium (Club Nose)

Depressive and hypochondriacal, there are chronic gastric and indigestion problems with weakness whenever a meal is delayed or missed. Not loners but the child is rather solitary and often alone in their own company, as long as there is someone else in the next room. There is a tendency to hypochondriacal preoccupations – especially concerned with illness. Other remedies which fear disease are *Lac. Caninum*, *Lil tig*, *Nit Ac*, *Nux vom*, *Phos Phos Ac*, *Sepia*, *Tril*.

Aconitum (Monkshood)

Restless, convinced that he or she is going to die, they may even predict the exact time of death. The fears are aggravated by shock of any form.

Infantile Hypochondriasis

Natrum Mur. (Sodium Chloride)

Hypochondriasis, but mainly centred about the intestines and bowels (indigestion and constipation).

Sepia (Ink of Cuttlefish)

Hypochondriasis centred around problems of portal and venous congestion, the child is liverish, with a poor circulation, flushed, and a tendency to retain fluid.

Infantile Passivity and Personality Disorders

Causes

These are usually known unless there is a history of an earlier physical or psychological trauma. One or both parents may be 'quiet' and/or subdued, too controlled or 'laid-back' upon themselves which has a negative effect on the child's personality development. The parents may favour a rigid, restrictive type of upbringing, rather than a more spontaneous approach which makes for a dull, subdued child. In many cases, there is a combination of genetic factors and a restrictive upbringing which creates the conditions for passivity to occur.

Symptoms

The child is best described as reluctant or tearful, holding back and too dependent, only rarely showing aggression or disagreeing, when they then may bully a younger weaker child, sometimes quite severely or secretly. In general they disobey in controlled moderation and are far too well-behaved and controlled. Fear of the reactions and disapproval of others, acts as a severe brake on spontaneous expressions and security.

Infantile Passivity and Personality Disorders

Remedies

Always try to prescribe the constitutional remedy for the child in high potency. For extreme passivity give *Pulsatilla* or *Lycopodium*. For disturbed, more aggressive personality disorders give *Nux. vom.* For an anxious, timid, withdrawn child consider *Silicea*. For a more obsessional controlling make-up consider *Arsenicum*. A fearful, unconfident personality may require *Phosphorus*.

Infantile Depression

Causes

The commonest cause is psychological damage in some form to the growing child's normal development which leads to feelings of rage, anger and frustration. Suppressed urges to break, fragment or destroy, may also lead to fear and a sense of guilt so that insecurity occurs at the same time. A sense of loss or alienation is common, with loneliness. In many cases there is a family history of depression. Where hereditary disposition is combined with an over-sensitive, vulnerable make-up, then even a minor psychological trauma may cause damage

126

and depression as an outcome, because of inability to adequately and openly deal with the feelings as they occur at the time. Unresolved grief and loss involving a parent, grandparent or a sibling is sometimes a factor, where the loss was unprepared for or not fully and adequately expressed at the time.

Damage to basic security, love and vulnerability undermines basic trust, reassurance and acceptance. The psychological needs for reassurance are increased. There may have been a flattening of the basic ego and confidence by rejection, sometimes physical and psychological hurts, pain and rejection.

Symptoms

These include fear, avoidance of others, even of friends and the absence of spontaneity or joy. In general they feel flat and down. Pain may be either psychological or physical with cramps, headache or 'stomach-ache'. Sometimes they take on the symptoms of an adult member of the family complaining of 'migraine' or a down or depressing day. Any change is a threat which puts them on guard, on the spot or feeling under scrutiny both at school and in the home. There is a reluctance to play competitive games, or indeed anything other than quiet, solitary occupations where they can be alone and in control of their thoughts and preoccupations. They feel unable to initiate, to participate or be involved except rarely when they forget themselves. Often bored, they find nothing interesting, except food and warmth. In severe cases, they are even disinterested in such creature comfort and lie listless in bed or on a chair, not wanting to do anything or to be involved. Suicide may sometimes be a risk when depression is severe, and may occur after being bullied by other children at a time when they feel inadequate, isolated and unable to find help from any source. Insomnia with nightmares is common and often the schoolwork suffers because of lack of interest and concentration, adding further to pressure and misery.

Remedies for Infantile Depression

Arsenicum (Arsenic Trioxide)

Cold and chilly even in mid-summer, the child is fearful (shivering), apathetic and discouraged too easily. Intellect is not affected although ideas and expressions are often rather rigid. There is a marked pride in appearance and a tendency to neat perfectionism. Exhibitionism and showing off are also common. At the same time as the apathy they are also restless, agitated and exhausted. There is often a combination of hopeless, fearful anxiety with restless agitation. Everything is controlled and the toys, bedroom and clothes are arranged in neat order. They usually dislike solitude, cold and night-time. Over-sensitive to both smells and touch, they resemble the child who needs *Nux vomica* but lack the imitable touchiness of this remedy.

Calc Phos.

See previous note.

Helleborus Niger. (Snow Rose)

Depression with fixed ideas, and a dull sluggishness to the point of stupor. Usually the child is too passive and withdrawn, lacking physical and psychological impetus and spontaneity.

Lachesis (Bushmaster Snake)

Alternating moods of excitement and depression, jealousy and pride may be a feature (*Hyoscy*) also talkative (*Stramonium* and *cocculus*). Religiose, with sadness. Worse on waking is characteristic, sad all morning, improving in the evening. Unable to concentrate, over-sensitive to closeness and to tight clothes.

18

Emotional Problems of Adolescence

Adolescent Depression

Causes

These are often obscure, difficult to explain and to verbalize. In general, the major depressive factors include problems like negative 'failure' imagery, guilt, grief, exams-pressure at school or university, peer-group pressures – including teasing or bullying, drugs abuse, either pharmaceutical or addictive. The actual cause, often dates back to infancy, with long-standing insecurity problems which are reactivated again in the teens. A change of environment, loss of friends and isolation may be a problem, from tension within the family, divorce and break-up, or a move to a new school or college which was psychologically unplanned. In a fragmented family, one or both parents, developing new areas of relationship and interest may no longer want the teenager with them. Lack of confidence and assertion, so that there are few friends or interests and closed-in attitudes may also be a cause of depression in a sensitive child who feels unwanted and unloved. Any new different environment can be a trauma if not well prepared for by open discussion. Other causes include physical illness – glandular fever, hepatitis, influenza, late onset of measles or chicken pox. Anxiety about the health of a sibling or parent, who is seen as vulnerable, at a time when omnipotent phantasies are predominant, may also trigger depressive problems. There may have been damage to self esteem by rejection, violence, or being rejected in front of others, causing a humiliating dependency. All of this may stimulate a sense of resentment, suppressed anger and revenge phantasies, causing guilt and fear, sense of weakness and depression.

Symptoms of Adolescent Depression

Feeling bored, irritable, can't be bothered, aggressive, no interests. There may be threatening behaviour – to leave home, to kill themselves or to give up a job or studies. They often feel a failure without drive, energy or determination. There is a depressive refusal to go out, to meet people and make friends. He or she may sit alone, glued to the television or locked inside a Walkman cassette player headphones. Both smoking and drinking may be excessive. Insomnia is common and adds to the general sense of jaded boredom, lack of energy and interest.

Recommended Remedies for Adolescent Depression

Naja (Cobra venom)

Dullness and extreme languor, preoccupied with and meditates on his or her weakness which is a major source of anxiety. Unable to resolve or mobilize a stalemate situation and to express themselves, feeling trapped and caught-up by it. Suicidal tendencies (*Aurum Met.*). Easily excitable with palpitations. Generally they are over-intense.

Sepia (Cuttle Fish)

Indifferent, flat, aggressive at the same time as being exhausted and fearful. Although irritable and intolerant, they are nevertheless better for a party, for rapid exercise and enjoy dancing and people once they can be persuaded to join in. They feel worse for thunder and at the end of the day because of fatigue.

Natrum Mur

Tearful, weak, clumsy, flaring-up into a temper easily, the main mood is one of depression, worse for consolation and other people in general cause extreme irritability. They seek out solitude. Insomnia, from an over-active mind, preoccupied with their problems. In general they lack confidence and are intolerant of contradiction or interruption. Depression at puberty in either sex. Memory is weak in most areas, except the resentful ones, which preoccupy them.

Medusa (Jelly Fish)

Indicated for a cross, silent and disinterested adolescent. Recommended in 200C potency, 4 doses. (Cp. *Sepia*, *Natrum mur*). Especially an adolescent remedy.

Anorexia Nervosa

Causes

Invariably the patient is female, usually over-sensitive, with a compulsive tendency to deal with all of life's problems and difficulties by swallowing them, leading to a deep sense of shame and self-hate generally. All feelings are dealt with in this way, at the same time as compulsive eating. Often a close relative is obese and forms a threat to their image and security. Often one parent has a weight problem and like the daughter, swings from compulsive eating or talking to dieting and a moody withdrawal.

Symptoms

There is a distorted, 'fat' self-image coupled with an inappropriate excessive fear of obesity. Weight loss may fall to a critical level, sometimes as low as to six stones or even less. Such low body weight levels are critical to normal physical functioning and lead to constipation, amenorrhoea, weakness or chill with loss of body fat. Vomiting may be provoked after eating, to lose more weight, or food may be regurgitated and hidden. But other times there are sudden uncontrollable and compulsive periods of devouring cakes, chocolate, crisps and sweets.

Recommended Remedies for Adolescent Anorexia Nervosa

Thuja (Tree of Life)

Fixed ideas with a grossly disturbed body image. There may be a history of never being well since vaccination. The body feels as if made of glass and there are a multitude of odd, bizarre hypochondriacal body preoccupations, the body image even distorted and elongated in one limb.

Cannabis Indica (Indian Hemp)

Dreamy and very talkative, time seems to pass too slowly (*Medorrhinum*, *Arg Nit*, *Nux Vom*). There is a sense of having a double (*Anacardium*, *Baptisia*, *Petroleum*, *Stamonium*).

Natrum Mur (Common Salt)

There is a much more depressive note to the anorexia. Especially note the tearfulness, the typical intolerance and the independence. Salt craving is common and they are either worse or better for being at the seaside.

Platina (The Metal Platinum)

There is a combination of pride, arrogance and egocentricity with a marked sense of superiority. Much of this, however, hides a well-defended position of failure and unconscious lack of confidence. Everything and everyone around seems smaller, but the body image is often felt to be gross, enlarged and unacceptable. Irritable and angry, there is malice and arrogance is characteristic.

Other Remedies to Consider Where The Body Feels Too Large Or Fat

Alumina   Usually worse on waking and all symptoms are aggravated at that time (also compare *Lachesis*, *Aesculis*, *Lycopodium*, *Sulphur*).

Hyoscyamus There is delirium and a tormented excitability.

Opium Passive and drowsy, they keep falling asleep. Constipation is severe.

Picric Acid A particularly good children's remedy with weakness of concentration and any form of learning.

Stramonium The disturbance of body image is also associated with moods of excitement and restlessness.

Adolescent Schizoid Illness

Causes

These are largely unknown. The roots of the disease may be viral or infective in origin, or due to an unknown metabolic disturbance within the brain cell physiology, possibly linked to a genetic factor. Psychological factors always play a major role in the illness and these do not seem to be secondary to other causes. It is still not clear how much these relate to possible physical causes, despite many years of international research in different centres.

Symptoms

These are usually vagueness, feelings of unreality, mistrust and fear. Hostility, insecurity and a variety of negatives are projected into others or outside situations causing suspicion and doubt. Weakness and uncertainty, preoccupation with ideas and vague phantasies, leads to delusions, sometimes of a sexual nature as well as severe problems of relating to others as the body is experienced as distorted, and initiative and control is felt to be at the command and suggestion of others – because so much of the self is thrust outside and into others.

Remedies

One side of the body feels alive, the other dead or buried – *Cannabis Indica*. The body seems blackened in colour – *Sulphur*. The body feels brittle and abnormally vulnerable – *Thuja*. The body is experienced as divided or split – *Petroleum*. The body feels scattered and in pieces – *Baptisia*. Generalized and vague, rather grandiose ideas – *Phosphorus*.

Adolescent Anxiety

Causes

Security is threatened often as a carry-over from a childhood anxiety state, with a continuation of lack of confidence, excessive vulnerability and attention-provoking ways. There may be sexual insecurity, fears and undisclosed problems with the opposite sex. Moody resentment may undermine relationships and cause problems of fear and tension. There are poor controls generally, and violence may occur in an intolerable situation – to have out and release at all costs creating further anxiety.

Symptoms

Impulsive, changing and changeable in everything. Fearful, imaginative, over-tense, jumpy, with mood swings of intense emotion. Preoccupied with details and the negative. Irritable, impulsive, weepy, demanding, resentful, with everything extreme and either excessive, over-intense or secretive and a phantasy rather than reality level. A tendency to be solitary and to avoid others, especially new contacts.

Recommended Remedies for Adolescent Anxiety States

Pulsatilla (Anemone Wind Flower)

Weak, variable, tearful, too passive, accepting and agreeable. The peace-maker, but on their own territory where they feel more secure and less vulnerable and with a smaller weak person, they can be very nasty, bullying and sadistic. This may account for some of the surface tearfulness and depression and the sense of vulnerability – a reaction to denied aggressive impulses.

Natrum Mur (Common Salt)

Never relaxed or themselves in any situation, nor able to fully participate or enjoy life. They are tearful, hopeless, depressed, often prematurely old or old-fashioned before they have been young. Sometimes they have never been a child, and have always had an 'old' look about them. Rigid in attitudes, irritable and hardened at an early age. They mainly want to be left to themselves. Immature intellectually and emotionally, the least enforced contact with others gives rise to an acute sense of inadequacy as well as irritation.

Lycopodium (Club Moss)

Bright, popular and attractive, there is a pseudo-maturity present and the company of older adults is constantly sought. Immature emotionally, they seek acceptance, reassurance, and lack of competition from older people with whom they seek to identify, in order to give them a temporary confidence and identity for use with their own peer groups and to impress. Hypochondriacal complaints are common, especially in the intestinal regions and chest regions. Clumsy and always too quick, never sensing a physical obstacle or hurdle, they inevitably spill the milk or fall over. Unreliable, almost every clumsy misfortune possible, seems to happen to them and this undermines confidence. Too quick and impulsive, yet they also have considerable social ease and skill with others. Their lack of confidence is covered up by adult, often impressive, name-dropping or pseudo-intellectual talk. Artistic, often with considerable real talent and ability and good at acting, their adult-identification defence prevents true growth and maturing and confidence from developing.

Phosphorus

Bright, flushing-up, self-conscious and self-aware to a painful degree, blushing is common. Outgoing, interested and caring, they enjoy the company of others, but lack confidence and need constant attention and reassurance. They are often highly artistic, gifted and sensitive teenagers.

Arsenicum

Cold, more rigid, controlled and calculating people, they tend to have over-active and restless personalities, chilly physically as well as emotionally. Intellectually bright, they are achievers and successful, hard-working young people who nevertheless quickly get exhausted. There is a tendency to be too well-dressed and fussy in their appearance. They are over-tidy in most areas, too rigid, which keeps them on the fringe of life, seeking to avoid or to impress others from a distance. There is fear of inadequacy, and failure. The controlled obsessional tendencies and lack of spontaneity makes every contact with others a tense situation and usually all closeness is carefully avoided.

19

Emotional Problems of Adults

Adult Anxiety

Causes

These are often a carry-over of adolescent insecurity or infantile attitudes of immaturity. Fear, over-caution, or attention-seeking demands undermine confidence and a more mature exchange of ideas and viewpoints. Such attitudes are often familiar, repetitive and run along familiar pathways and patterns, creating recurrent problems and difficulties rather than challenges or opportunities. A rejecting or over-controlling upbringing may have caused damage to personality development by adults seeking to impose their own values and ideas upon a vulnerable developing mind, causing limitations and a build-up of resentment which is difficult to dispense in later years. In general, such controls seek to reduce the threat of others bringing or questioning often narrow, unthought-out beliefs and blinkered attitudes. Psychological hurt, grief, loss and weakened experiences of loving and closeness all impose a distorted attitude or a defensiveness which distorts all later adult relationships into a mould of either limitation or rejection. Where there has been a recent blow to self-esteem, pride or security, this may also be a reactivating factor to earlier traumas and release infantile anxiety from that time.

Symptoms

These may be either physical or psychological. Typically they manifest as a general sense of tension and inability to relax. There is often a vague sense of foreboding, or restlessness with spasm or irritability, sometimes pain, as part of the physiological malaise which occurs. Diarrhoea, constipation or spasm may occur in any area of the body, day or night. Nervous eczema is also common. Frequency of urination, nausea, sweating, palpitations and loss of appetite are common because they undermine sleep or relaxation and because they can also court sympathy and concern as well as familiar and protective adult attitudes towards them.

Recommended Remedies for Adult Anxieties

Aconitum

Extreme fear is the key-note – fear of everything, especially of shadows, or some vague indefinable something, unknown and undesirable. There is fear of fear itself. The anxiety is felt to be irrational but is also uncontrollable with an overwhelming sense of anguish. Over-intensity of the personality makes every experience too much, too acute, or experienced in too great a detail. Each event is given too much meaning or significance. Loss of confidence is marked, often acutely so, and especially after acute fear or shock. Attitudes are totally rigid and they are convinced of the reality of all beliefs, convictions and fears (*Nat mur*). Fears are constant, leading to nervous agitation, worse for music which cannot be tolerated in any form. Palpitations are common.

Nux Vomica

The ideal remedy for the over-stretched executive who cannot delegate and is exhausted from trying to do too much. Irritable, a worrier and much too quickly involved, they fly off the handle into tempers and then down again just as quickly. There is only short fuse tolerance. Easily despondent and defeated, he or she is resentful of interference. Commonly associated with gastric problems especially with a history of duodenal or peptic ulcer, spasm, heart-burn or hiatus hernia are common. Blood pressure, heart problems such as angina pectoris may occur, although they are often surprisingly fit. In any sport they play a hard competitive game. More chronic than *Aconitum* but less visibly agitated and fearful, they are very controlled and tense, keeping things in until they boil over with sudden blow-outs of feelings. Control and tension is reflected in the lack of relaxation and a healthy relaxed tone in muscles so that any quick effort or movement may catch them off-balance and lead to a chronic tennis-elbow or low-back condition. They drive themselves as they drive others – excessively and without tolerance. When they drive a vehicle, it is usually too fast and they take risks. Angry and intolerant at the wheel because of the faults and erratic behaviour of others they rarely criticize themselves. They may be involved in uncontrollable arguments with other motorists, to the point of threats of violence.

Causticum (Hydrated Caustic, Lime and Bisulphite of Potash)

There is depressive anxiety, worse in the evening or at twilight. They dislike being alone and there are overwhelming feelings of sympathy for the problems of others, taking their pains and difficulties into themselves excessively, both moved and upset by them. Easily irritated, but, at other moments silent and moody, they cannot think or concentrate. Note the improvement for warm rain (*Ruta*) and the aggravation at 3–4.00 a.m. They feel worse for thinking about their 'problems'. Note the commonly associated weakness, exhaustion, cramps and the tendon contractures, especially of the hands and feet.

Secale (Ergot)

Depressive fear and anxiety with irrational impulses to throw themselves into water. Lack of concentration. The agitation is at times very severe.

Sulphur

Too easily excited and enthusiastic by a vague plan or idea which is not realistically based, they lack the fervour, drive, or the resentment of *Nux vom*. Weak, often thin and unhealthy looking, they feel irritable and unwell because they lack drive. There is a great deal of talking but little is usually accomplished and often their favourite occupation is eating anything and everything, at any time of the day, provided that food and atmosphere is cool and not over-heated. The choice of food is usually unwise and accounts for the unhealthy skin and a loose, offensive bowel motion. When eating they like to talk about themselves and their plans, rarely listening or very concerned with other people's needs. In general talk is everything and action is put off until tomorrow. Untidy in mind, ideas and appearance, they are quickly tearful and exhausted with no reserves of energy. There is little insight into the phantasy nature of the speculative, philosphic talk, but they are not unachievers and this is usually blamed on bad luck or circumstance. Their basic plans and ideas usually considered to be above those of others (*Platina*). There is also an uneasy anxiety, quickly denied by more eating or ideas talk.

Adult Depression

Causes

Inseparable from the reasons for adult anxiety, there is often a recurrence of a long-standing earlier problem or conflict which has never been fully resolved in the past. The actual origins are often infantile and they may have mild, even severe depression at that time. Typical infantile causes are sibling (brother or sister) rivalry, an acute loss or grief experience, feelings of another being preferred, or the favourite one, feeling unloved. There may be a reactivation of these earlier conflicts,

144

triggered off by a happening which floods the senses with intense emotion and fatigue. For many, depression is an old and endlessly repetitive theme that has never been properly resolved because it has never been fully acknowledged and consciously or openly admitted. In this way insight is either partial or minimal. There may also be a general tendency to cling to former worn-out attitudes of clinging dependency, fear and past preoccupations or regrets which drag-down and limit growth and maturation from experience and contact because of inappropriate guilt.

Symptoms

A vague, dragged-down sense with boredom, with lack of drive and poor general health. Any temporary 'better' feeling may be brief, inappropriate or excessive and self-destructive in some way, which does not really match the true reasons for exhilaration or the energy and drive. A deep trough with low thoughts of failure and futility usually follows and is accompanied by an almost complete absence of energy and drive.

Recommended Remedies

Aurum Met (Gold)

Depressed, they can't be roused from despair by reassurance or encouragement. Quick tempered, with marked resentment and indignation (cp. *Staphisag*, *Nux. vom*), egocentricity is marked with conviction of failure. Obsessed by guilt, they become preoccupied with determined impulses to destroy themselves. Despair is linked to a wish to be alone, weeping and sighing, desiring death and making plans for it. Over-sensitive to strong tastes, smell and noise, they are always worse for colds or draught. Note the common accompanying cardiac symptoms of palpitations, extra-systoles and raised blood pressure. Better generally for music and attention from others.

The following remedies also have suicidal impulses.

Alumina Especially at the sight of blood or a knife.

Arg. Nit Obsessional desires to fling themself from an open window into space.

Capiscum Nostalgia with suicidal impulses.

Naja Wants to commit suicide because of hypochondriacal anxiety about the heart.

Nat. Sulph There is a constant battle waged against suicidal impulses.

Nux. Vom Suicidal impulses which are the out-come of a sudden irritation, provoking violent desires with overwhelming temper and rage.

China (Peruvian Bark, Quinine)

Weakness with exhaustion (cp. *Carbo Veg*, *Arsenicum*). The mind is overactive in spite of exhaustion. Ideas follow one another without a pause, preventing sleep and much-needed rest. Over-sensitive to an extreme degree, physically and emotionally, there is an apathetic, indifferent, silence, lack of confidence, drive and determination. Reluctant to move, they seem quite unable to find their way out of the apathy and languor. Hypochondriacal, crying or groaning with com-plaints, yet also flying into rage and anger of a homicidal murderous degree and at other times to impulses of suicide.

146

Lilium Tig. (Tiger Lily)

They are so depressed that they can hardly think or concentrate. Timid, they want to cry, and are worse for consolation (*Nat. mur*). The whole pattern of syntax and phrases is lost with blocks of words or ideas forgotten completely. Worse for concentration, they often have to think of something else before they can recover the 'lost' phrase or thought. At times they feel sure they are going mad. They must always be busy, agitated and in a hurry and cannot relax (cp. *Arg. Nit*, *Merc. Med*, *Nat. Mur*, *Nux. vom*, *Sulph.*). Violent, irritable outbursts of temper, rage and anger are typical of the remedy.

Murex (Purple Fish)

This is especially a valuable menopausal remedy. There is sadness with anxiety and dread or fear. There are hysterical tendencies and generally they are very tense. Libido and sexual drive is increased as they are over-sensitive generally. Intolerant of being touched or exaimed (*Kali Carb.*).

Nitric Acid

Prostrated and indifferent by depression which is worse at night. Tearfulness and obstinate is characteristic and they won't be consoled (*Nat. Mur*). Full of fears or hypochondriacal, they are often vindictive. There is relief from movement and travel (*Tub. Bov*, *Rhus tox*). Very sensitive to chill and draughts.

Psorinum

Sad, hopeless and suicidal with an overall attitude of negative pessimism. There are many fixed delusional ideas of guilt during the day and in dreams at night. An absence of joy (*Sepia*). Obsessional thoughts are also common (*Arsen*), feeling convinced of their overall failure and unworthiness – although in fact and in reality everything outwardly is going well. Irritable, they want to be left alone (*Nat Mur.*). Dislike of water and showering and bathing is marked and characteristic (*Sulphur*). In general of offensive appearance, neglected, untidy and unkempt, they are always better for lying down and worse for the least activity because every movement causes fatigue.

Thuja (Tree of Life)

Depression with agitation, anxiety and excitability. Intellectual weakness. Every symptom is worse since vaccination and never well since that time. Over-impressionable, especially music causes weeping (cp. *Aconitum*, *Graphites*, *Sabina*). There are many often bizarre, fixed-ideas, for example that they have a live animal in the abdomen (cp. *Crocus*, *Sulphur*). They also feel under the influence of a Superior Power (*Anacardium*) and that the body is fragile and made of glass (*Lachesis*), or a strange person is by their side, or that body and self are divided. (Cf. *Opium*, *Platina*.)

Zincum met.

Both memory and concentration are weak, the individual feels tired and forgetful. They frequently repeat comments or questions before replying, as distracted and not really listening. Vague in understanding, they are unable to pinpoint what is said or it feels just beyond grasp.

Nervous prostration with depression is common. They feel far away but then suddenly wake up and reply with a start. There is great variability of mood, ranging from humour to sadness, calm to rage. Hypochondriasis is a feature, also boredom with everything, especially intellectual work and studies. They are over-sensitive to noise with a paralytic weakness of limbs as of meningitis, polio or multiple sclerosis. Weakness with tremor and spasm of isolated muscle groups as in Motor Neurone Disease (cp. *Arsen. Cimicifugea, Crocus, Cuprum, Ignatia, Mygale, Stramonium, Tarant, Veratrum Viride, Zigia*). Note the diagnostically restless fidgety feet.

Agoraphobia (Adult)

Causes

There is an underlying fear of making a break from a static, closed, psychological situation which is 'safe' but also frustrating and unfulfilling. Admitting needs or coming out into the open with feelings is difficult to express, although this also leads to vulnerability. A typical and largely unconscious conflict of clinging to the safety of the edges and the periphery of situations and life in general is usual, at the same time contrasting with an urge to come out into the open, both physically and psychologically with needs, aims and feelings. All of this leads to conflict, anxiety and to phobia or fear, avoidance and control marked in specific situations – in case there is loss of control. There is a wish to be free and more open conflicting with wanting to stay safe. Ideas, feelings, life in general and sexuality all have to run this same gauntlet of wanting greater freedom of expression and a tendency to stay remote, hidden, more in the shade. They feel run down by their lack of initiative and holding-back, self-destructive attitudes, which also cause intense frustration and anger. The infantile origins are shown by childish attitudes in many areas as repression attempts to control the whole of life and to keep the personality at an infantile level.

Fear of open spaces, of not being able to get back, of being caught on a motorway, queue or traffic jam is common and reflects feelings of being unable to flee and being trapped, as well as a wish to be held and prevented from going back into the old patterns and conflicts. Such patterns give little to satisfy or fulfil and lead to only greater urges to break-out, which intensifies the anxiety and fear.

Recommended Remedies

Aconitum

Always worse for cold, dry winds, at night towards midnight. In a warm room. For wine and stimulants. For tobacco smoke. For music, noise, light. For fear, emotion of any form. It is better for fresh air, rest, after perspiration.

Argentum nit

The remedy is worse for heat in any form, at night, for sweet foods – causing flatulence and indigestion, period times, after eating, for lying down on the right side. It is better for fresh, cool air, local pressure and burping.

Gelsemium

This is aggravated by wet, cold, damp weather, thinking of their problems (*Calc. phos.*), tobacco. It is better for fresh air, stimulants generally, passing urine, leaning forward.

Adult Paranoid Illness

Causes

The reasons behind an adult paranoid illness are usually obscure and unknown, the processes of onset, often slow, subtle and drawn-out over months or years. In some cases the illness follows an acute trauma or shock in a personality which was previously over-controlled, rigid or obsessional in attitudes as well as brittle and vulnerable. In some cases the controlling was very marked with obvious obsessional components to the personality.

Case History I A man of 40, developed an acute paranoid illness after surgical amputation of his right arm which was crushed when the scaffolding he was erecting collapsed. Prior to this there has been a long-standing obsessional tendency, and a rather paranoid, suspicious personality make-up, largely hidden by a combination of heavy social drinking in the evenings and a tendency to keep a 'safe' distance from other people.

Case History II A man of 55, with a long-standing severe chronic obsessional problem, suddenly began running into the street, knocking at a neighbour's door in the middle of the night and feeling acutely persecuted and attacked. This followed the pressures in the office preparing figures for the financial year and having them audited. The imagined pressures and deadlines of the audit were turned into an acute persecutory pressure situation which changed the chronic obsessional state into a more serious and acute paranoid one.

Symptoms

These vary considerably, but in general they feel isolated or ostracized by others, 'got at' and criticized or different and disliked. The feelings of suspicion and resentment may be of a controlled violent nature. There is a tendency to blame others, their plots and schemes, for any limitations or problems and which they feel makes them an innocent victim. The remarks of others may be heard as obscene and of a sexual nature. References to homosexuality or impotency are common and refer to unconscious preoccupations in this area as well as guilt.

Recommended Remedies for Adult Paranoid Illness

Aconitum

There is great violence within a delusional pattern of fear and convictions of imminent death or destruction.

Cannabis indica (Hemp)

Excited, talkative and changeable (cp. *Hyoscyamus*, *Lachesis*, *Stramonium*), this alternates with moods of laughter and tears. Time passes too slowly (cp. *Alumina*, *Arg. nit.*, *Med.*, *Nux.*). A multitude of ideas crowd-in upon the mind preventing effective concentration and comprehension. At times exhilarated with a wealth of wonderful ideas, phantasies or hallucinations; they seem to exist on two planes at the same time. The mind is full of unfinished, unending and irresolvable ideas, phantasies and theories. Auditory hallucinations such as bells, voices, music in an ecstatic cacaphony of confusion is common.

Lachesis (Bushmaster snake venom)

Self-conscious with feelings of hate, envy, murderous revenge and cruelty. Jealousy and suspicion are particularly marked. People are felt to be talking about them or whispering, trying to damage or mis-represent their reputation. The family is felt to be plotting to get them locked away. Fears of being poisoned or that the food is interfered with in some way. There are dreams of being dead, that a strange power influences them. Voices give commands, tell them to confess, that they are being pursued. Religiose or secret sexual preoccupations crowd in upon them, worse in the morning or after sleep.

Sulphur

There is a peculiar philosophical mania of unreality (Kent) with self-centredness marked and an unresolvable philosophical rambling. Religiose, with delusions of importance, they feel that others fail to understand the significance and importance of their system, knowledge or genius.

20

Emotional Problems of the Elderly

Depression of the Elderly

Causes

These include loneliness, grief and mourning reactions, physical pain, vertigo or arthritis. Social isolation, deafness, loss or diminished sight as with a cataract, can also cause isolation or confusion. All of these may create a subtle personality change so that people and events are misunderstood or misrepresented. Senility and ageing can also lead to confused ideas, especially when combined with an acute infection. The physical limitation of being confined to bed for several weeks after a fracture, or sometimes where it has been necessary to give treatment in a different and strange environment for a time – a hospital or nursing home can also cause depression. The sudden unexpected loss of a friend or neighbour may lead to shock and fear with emotional disorientation. Such feelings are far more intense when the loss is of a partner or spouse.

Symptoms

These include loss of confidence, insomnia, fear and hypochondriasis. There may be physical problems too, as loss of appetite or confusion leads to neglect with hypothermia or lack of warm and balanced meals. In general there is loss of interest in food, hygiene and exercise as well as of life in general. Constipation is common and may become a source of worry and preoccupation. Tearfulness, suicidal ideas and suicidal determination may occur in acute and severe cases.

Recommended Remedies in Depression of the Elderly

Anacardium orientale (Marking Nut)

Indicated when weak-minded, feeble or over-intense. The least effort or strain causes pain, anxiety and a migrainous type of headache. They live in a dream-like state of unawareness and unreality. Loss of memory is often severe, and they spend hours trying to recapture and recall a name. Hypochondriacal, they are also spiteful and irritable at times, full of contradictions or suspicious, with loss of confidence in most areas. Unable to take a decision or make up their mind they are uncertain about everything. There are many contradictory impulses. Hallucinated, at times hearing voices, they feel they have a double because of senile dissociation and a break-down of personality (cp. *Baptisia* – where the self is in bits and trying to integrate them together; *Cannabis indica* – feels split or has a double, *Petroleum* – a double sleeps by his or her side in the bed, *Stramonium* – feels

155

confused, in bits, split, has a double or that part of his mind and identity is not there – missing or absent). Note the typical and diagnostic desire for swearing, using violent, gross language (cp. *Stramonium* – which swears constantly, often continuously). Note the important diagnostic modality that all symptoms are better for eating and/or during the digestive process. They are also usually less confused at meal-times.

Baryta carb. (Carbonate of Baryta)

The remedy for senility and second childhood where there are depressive features. There is timidity and fear of strangers with inability to concentrate or to think clearly. Ideas are confused and they are depressed about minor, unimportant issues with misplaced scruples and a poor memory (cp. *Sulphur* with a poor memory for names and can only recall remote early happenings, not the most recent events; *Lycopodium* – forgets the significance of words and letters, using them wrongly with faults and lapses in writing; *Nux moschata* – a weak, exhausted memory, forgets words and letters; *Anacardium* – can't remember the right word for what they want to say). They seem to create anxiety over problems of their own making, without reason, purely from a broken-down intellectual process dominated by misplaced imagination and phantasy.

Confusional States of the Elderly

Causes

Any sudden shock, either emotional or physical. An acute physical illness with a high temperature, as occurs in influenza, or bronchitis of the elderly may cause confusion. In a mild form it is common after any change in the familiar environment, particularly any sudden unplanned or unexpected move to a hospital, clinic or nursing home. This always causes some confusion, but when associated with an illness or debilitated state, is much more severe. In the elderly states of disorientation, regression and confusion are more marked than at any other stage of life and this is why confusion is common and often intense.

Symptoms

Restlessness, rapid shallow thought, with confused unrelated ideas, often linking back to the past, full of suspicion and danger as a reflection of their own fragmented self and the heightened sense of vulnerability that is experienced as a result. Insomnia, over-activity and anxiety are all common with a high level of tension and an inability to be at peace.

Recommended Remedies in Confusional States of the Elderly

Ambra grisea (Morbid Secretion of the Whale)

There is a state of premature senility, with sadness, trembling and weakness. The mind jumps from one subject and idea to another, not able to answer to what is said in a related way. Flights of talk and phantasy occur without logic or sometimes syntax. Talkative and impulsive, there is a confused dreamy state, especially over past hurts and grievances. The premature breakdown of the intellec-

157

tual processes may follow severe shock – the collapse of a business, breakdown of a relationship or a state of severe grief (*Ignatia*). There is alternating depression with irritability. Usually the mental state is worse in the mornings with confusion and dullness, at times with severe confusion.

Belladonna (Deadly Nightshade)

There is a violent and disturbed agitated destructive state of mind, the face red and suffused, the skin hot, flushed or congested. Intensity of the mental state causes anger, even fury and they may become either manic or stuperose, with auditory and visual sensory disturbances. Nightmares are common and usually very disturbed.

Nux moschata (Nutmeg)

There is weakness, unable to think or concentrate. Changeable and inconsistent, the moods vary from sadness to great joy, laughter or tears (cp. *Alumina*, *Ignatia*, *Platina*, *Crocus*, *Zincum*). Weakness of memory, forgetting what they want to say (cp. *Anacardium*, *Baryta carb.*, *Camphor*, *Cannabis Indica*, *Lachesis*, *Nat. mur.*, *Mercurius*, *Sulphur*). Unable to concentrate, think or to assemble ideas in any order that may be coherently expressed (cp. *Anacardium*, *Kreosotum*, *Lachesis*, *Nat. mur.*, *Mercurius*).

Onosmodium (False Gromwell)

Weakness with prostration, lack of concentration and co-ordination. Impotence, loss of memory, migraine.

Opium (Poppy)

Sluggish, painless states of inactivity, wanting to be alone (*Nat. mur.*). Fear, at other times feeling at peace wanting nothing or nobody – just to be left undisturbed. Euphoric, almost to the point of being stuperose and drowsy. The exalted ideas and visions are at times like a vivid nightmare. Visual delusional phantasies (cp. *Lachesis* – snakes or being strangled; *Stramonium* – animals of a violent nature are hiding in the corner of the room; *Cannabis Indica*, – confusion of both time and space; *Arsenicum* – fear of death and doesn't want to be left alone; *Calc. carb.* – terrified of phantasies that occur as soon as he closes the eyes).

Petroleum (Crude Rock-oil)

Irritable to the point of violence and over-sensitive. Nausea is a feature and they are too quickly moved and hurt – even for a trifle (*Nux*). Lose their way in familiar situations. Over-impressionable and hypochondriacal, the least symptom of malaise is interpreted as a sign of incurable disease. Hallucinations – his or her double lies beside them in bed. Exhausted and worn-out, often prematurely. Especially the eyes are weak.

Strychnine (Alkaloid of *Nux vom*)

Explosive nervous excitement with spasm and restless. Irritability, throws his or her body around, often dangerously. Cramping pains with sudden jerky movements (*Lyc*).

Cocculus (Indian Cockle)

There is a typical picture of irritable prostration and weakness (cp. *Phosphoric ac.*). Time passes too quickly. Slow to understand, the mind feels empty to the point of idiocy. Confusion is such that he or she cannot find the words to express themself, the tongue feels as if paralysed. Obsessionally repeats a phrase or idea and also irritable, the least contradiction or command, causes an outburst of temper. They can also be serene and smiling with an empty mind, but exhausted in body and mind from anxiety and loss of sleep. Tremor of hands, with vertigo or nausea. All symptoms are worse from movement travel and insomnia (cp. *Causticum*, *Cuprum*, *Ignatia*, *Nitric ac.*).

Anxiety States of the Elderly

Causes

Any break with routine and familiar patterns causes fear in an insecure personality. The symptoms may follow an actual physical assault, as after an attack or mugging, but more commonly they follow an imagined, phantasized or feared situation. The state of heightened emotion may follow an actual loss of someone close or significant, but often it is because of an imagined state of isolation, loss or being abandoned and not able to cope, because they feel too dependent and vulnerable. Sometimes the anxiety follows a quarrel or row, perhaps the ending of a relationship or friendship after many years without a previous overt disagreement. In many cases, the causes are unclear and never revealed, because neither emotions nor

160

feelings are given sufficient time or space to come up to the surface.

Symptoms

There is a trembling agitation with anguish, palpitations, and an inability to relax, unable to rest or sleep. Infantile fears of the dark or of a sudden noise at night is also common. Tearful, withdrawn, housebound, imaginative or fearful, excessive emotions, adds to the underlying anxiety, sometimes with a delusional intensity.

Recommended Remedies in Anxiety States of the Elderly

Phosphorus

Restless and tired yet always better for sleep and rest (an afternoon nap), they are depressed as well as indifferent to those around (*Sepia*). Tearful, irritable, often resentful and angry at fate or the system. They are tired and exhausted with life, unable to sleep as their mind is over-active. They cannot relax as they are so fearful and anguished. There is fear of an accident or some disaster happening – like a fall which would make them dependent and less mobile. The future seems sombre and one of despair. Worse in the evening as there is more time for depressive thinking to occur. Full of palpitations, extrasystoles and pulse irregularities which cause anxiety. All symptoms are worse for thunder, lightning and a storm (cp. *Calcarea*, *Cyclamen*, *Lil. tig.*, *Nux vom.*). There is also fear of being alone, abandoned or left. They are often on the brink of senility. All symptoms are worse and aggravated by noise, excitement, music, the dark, being alone or the threat of it.

Pulsatilla (Anemone, Wind Flower)

Tearful, passive, over-dependent, lacking confidence, they are changeable and unpredictable. Sad and over-sensitive, there is always an aggravation caused by heat or being alone.

Kali carb. (Potassium Carbonate)

Over-sensitivity is marked, especially to draughts of cold air or psychologically by any misunderstood comment or remark. Fearful and irritable, they are intolerant of being left alone causing severe fear. Never at peace with themselves or at rest in their mind (*Nat. mur.*). They feel worse from 3–5.00 a.m., often waking with fear and anxiety. The lack of confidence is variable and unpredictable. Apathetic and unable to concentrate or find the right words, the bed also feels as if it is collapsing or caving-in – perhaps an external representation of just how weak their mind feels.

Lycopodium (Club Moss)

Sensitive and artistic, yet fearful and usually worse in the early evening from 4–8.00 p.m. with an increase of anxiety and depression. Emotional with little confidence, especially for anything new, they fear a public appearance, meeting, appointment, or any visit to an unfamiliar area. There is a common sense of overwhelming dread and with a weakness, sense of failure – indeed conviction of it. Often they sit quiet, withdrawn and silent.

Delusional States of the Elderly

Causes

Sometimes the outcome of premature ageing or senility of unknown cause, it may also stem from familial or genetic roots. There may have been a sudden emotional shock at a critical stage in a vulnerable personality or a loss may have provoked acute feelings of vulnerability and the re-emergence of infantile fears lying dormant since childhood. There may also have been a strong forceful partner over the years so that fears of failure and of not coping well, were not seen or talked about, because they took charge and organized everything throughout the marriage. Such feelings only surfaced after many years, following a stage of acute grief, because they had never been admitted or acknowledged during the early years together.

Symptoms

Fear, persecution, vulnerability, hallucinations or delusions, sometimes of a sexual nature, with ideas of reference. The body feels odd, strange or changed in some way, with peculiar and 'different' areas of pain or distortion, as if containing a part of someone else. Bizarre patterns of behaviour may be the result of such delusional thinking which also has an infantile aspect to it, which clearly demonstrates the roots and origins of the problem.

Recommended Remedies in Delusional States of the Elderly

Recommended remedies to consider are
Hyoscyamus – Fear of being poisoned, or that the partner is unfaithful.

Kali brom. – That they have been singled out for divine vengeance.

Arsenicum – A sense of being watched.

Lac caninum – They are surrounded by snakes.

Belladonna – He or she sees ghosts, or dogs.

Mercurius – There are delusions of sexual interference, for example that things are creeping into the vagina.

Lachesis – Paranoid delusions are strong and they experience themselves under a powerful external influence.

Platina – Feels that he or she is divided or cut in two and that devils are present and surrounding them.

Thuja – Feels there is a live animal in the abdomen.

Cicuta – Thinks he or she is a child again.

Lycopodium – Full of childish phantasies.

Aconitum – Convictions that they are about to die.

Kali brom. – Fear of murdering spouse or child (also of value in puerperal states).

China – Delusions of persecution generally.

Cannabis indica – Feels transparent, floating and in another world.

Hypochondriasis of the Elderly

Causes

In general this is caused by a disturbed personality make-up where insecurity, fear and anxiety reflect the ageing process and a long-standing feeling of inadequacy and insecurity.

Symptoms

These are nearly always connected with the bowels and constipation, with anxiety about becoming

164

totally blocked, never functioning again, or developing a fatal incurable illness as a result.

There is a preoccupation with aperients, diet, laxatives and how to get their sluggish intestine moving again. But the problem is rarely resolved and the many different aperients tried only aggravate the difficulty. Anxiety and the intensity of their mental state is the most powerful cause of the constipation problem which reflects a sluggish state of mind. Other areas of preoccupation are of being paralysed, or falling and breaking a bone, cancer or heart problems. Sometimes they fear developing a more vague condition which will lead to incapacity or dependency. The individuals themself is often remarkably fit and there are little real grounds for the underlying anxiety and misery.

Recommended Remedies in Hypochondriasis of the Elderly

That they have heart disease – *Lac. caninum*, *Aurum met*.

The body is rotting or full of worns – *Cannabis indica*.

Their stomach is rotting – *Ignatia*.

The genital organs are distorted – *Sabadilla*.

The face is distorted, especially the nose or lip – *Glonoin*.

Their body feels dead – *Anacardium*, *Apis*.

That they have cancer – *Veratrum alb*.

Their body is diseased and incurable – *Stramonium*.

21

Anguish and Anxiety

Anguish is a philosophical, 'outside', position of modern man, to some extent increased by our stressed, pressurized world but generally universal and inevitable to some degree.

It is not an emotional illness and should not be seen as such, although the manifestations of existential uncertainty, the questioning of role, meaning and the purpose of life may give rise to symptoms which have a superficial resemblance to psychological problems and there can be overlap at times. Where the universal problem of existential doubt and uncertainty is not admitted and contained it gives rise to secondary anxiety, panic, fear, depression or irritability. These are usually treated at a superficial level, and not as the purely secondary manifestations of a deeper problem which is not immediately resolvable. Where there is no structure, faith, confidence, or belief to contain the uncertainties, there is the danger that their outer manifestations become confused with neurotic ones, and that tranquillizers or anti-depressants are heavily prescribed, leading to a chronic problem or failure to relieve the problem in any way.

Where there is a problem of anguish the person

feels 'out-of-true', isolated, unrelated or unable to relate to others – 'out of character' in everything. He or she feels unborn, not in harmony with their environment, the world as it is and as they are living their lives, with nothing much in common with others. Their lives seem more of a shadow of any real expression of their true self, in behaviour, ideals, expectations and life-style. In many ways everything feels wrong, the major symptom of malaise, of indefinable origin, usually long-standing and sometimes dating back to an event like a move from the country to the town in childhood or later. It is difficult to 'talk' to anyone about existential anguish, because in a sense there is nothing 'wrong', and there are 'no' problems. Friends and family say that he or she has every-thing they need to be happy – but in spite of them, there is a general absence of joy, and unhappiness is the commonest symptom.

In many ways, life feels like an unreal existence, something out of a fairy tale. Sometimes it is so unreal that it feels unbelievable and impossible that it could be true. It is not the Emperor who is unclothed and parading through the town, but the population as a whole, in a kind of naked denial of truth, reality, depth, awareness and knowing. Everyone says that they are alright and that he or she is too, that there is really nothing wrong – that there are no problems. It feels almost as if the whole of life is a kind of delusional existence yet this is no schizoid problem. There seems to be a collective collusion to prove that everything is alright, and that if you continue to wear the clothes of doubt (existential), uncertainty or sensitivity, then you are the odd one out and in danger of becoming sick and ill.

Being at odds with others creates its own position of doubt, uncertainty and isolation. Friends say why don't you have a valium or a sleeping tablet – we all do, it will do you no harm. The doctor recommends a tranquillizer – 'I take one when I feel down, like you, I give them to my family – they will do you no harm'. But he doesn't want either drugs or tranquillizers, doesn't feel 'ill' in that way, the anguish is one of uncertainty and not knowing, not the tension of fear and anxiety.

It is like the gynaecologist who says – 'You are over 40, you don't want any more children or you are not likely to have any now anyway – so why do you need to keep your uterus?' Others are quite happy – the women in the ward are not complaining, so why should you be the odd one out and want to keep and retain your uterus or breast. No one seems to understand that it is a part of her – of her intrinsic femininity, that it matters, that she is not just a collection of parts or bits to be removed or replaced at random without feeling deeply about it.

Guilt is artificially introduced because friends and the doctors say that there is nothing really wrong, no reason to be unhappy. He or she feels that as we have everything, we should be happy and contented. 'Please God that I should have your problems and tribulations', was the reply of a close friend to one of my patients.

In spite of the comfort which success brings and the convenience, these may also have no real meaning. The individual feels almost nauseated or saturated by them, so much so that a chronic state of nausea, with loss of appetite and disinterest may arise externally, and be quite refractory to all attempts to cure it or to remove the symptoms. (Cf. *Cocculus*, *Sepia*, *Nux vom.*)

Nothing has real appeal or great interest – especially where it involves things, activity, buying or moving. Everything seems jaded – but they are not truly depressed in terms of a depressive illness. Depression is quite secondary to the underlying problem. Another car, a larger house, a holiday in Spain gives little joy or excitement – friends say that she is spoiled and just doesn't appreciate all the family is trying to do for her which adds to the guilt and feelings of reproach. The usual response to any of the above suggestions is usually a flat one.

All of this leads to a powerful sense of isolation, from friends and family, although the 'motions' of a relationship are carried out and general contact with others may give a feeling of temporary improvement provided that it has been a real contact with a sharing rather than a superficial skirmish. The common and usual diagnosis and treatment is one of depression which is easy to make, but largely incorrect and not helpful because the unhappiness is of a deeper cause and level. There may be complaints of vertigo because they feel unattached to anything and anybody – like a lost soul, which adds to the feelings of being unsure of themselves.

Case History I

A woman of 76 came with degenerative vertigo, the husband senile and permanently in hospital. She lived alone and was physically and mentally young for her years. She felt giddy night and day at any time. All physical investigations had proved negative. There was considered to be a degenerative change in the inner ear balance centre. But the problem was very variable, there were days when she was fine and all symptoms absent or minimal. On other days when severe, they made life a misery. She was worse for movement, stress and emotion of any kind and always better for being absorbed. She had recently spent an evening watching television, felt totally absorbed and enjoyed it as she had not enjoyed anything for weeks. She began to feel more adhered, more together, better and stronger. When I see her, she never feels giddiness at the time, can talk and relate to me and feels better for it. Just a lonely old woman – you may say. She certainly looks forward to a visit, but is made worse for sedatives or tranquillizers and cannot take them because of side-effects and drowsiness. After a consultation, she feels more attached, less all over the place, more integrated, with more confidence, is less lonely and less unsure of herself. Usually this lasts for several days with the vertigo less acute, until there is return of the symptoms.

Case History II

A woman of 30 was married with two children – a young baby and a boy of three – described as difficult and demanding. She doesn't like being a mother to 'young' children and resents the lack of freedom yet feels guilty about the feelings. All her friends love and like *their* children, why should she feel different? She is embarrassed by her son when he is naughty and difficult and feels guilty about it and that this is a reflection on her and her 'bad' upbringing or mothering which is the real cause of it. Yet she does not seem to really believe this either. She needs to get out more from the home, away from the children and hates it there, yet also feels that she should both like and enjoy it. If she smacks the boy, the baby cries and she feels worse. When friends come, they all have children and there is no *real* conversation because they keep interrupting and leaping about. She feels guilty, depressed, and a failure if she admits that it is not all lovely and ideal or that she hates it all at times.

She cannot be herself – the key-note of her anguish position. She says she 'rattles around inside herself', constantly complaining to her friends and husband all the time yet feeling guilty about it, unable to be herself or to be angry properly. The family say she needs a break or more help. But she feels caught up in a situation where one must conform to the model of a happy wife and mother – but 'it is just not her or that rosy'. She was not in a state of puerperal depression, there were no neurotic relationship problems, and the basic temperament is a warm attractive one with no history of trauma and she relates and expresses herself well. Another tired housewife and mum – you may say who needs more rest, leisure and support, or is it a position of anguish which cannot be expressed for a variety of reasons?

Her basic anguish is one which is very common to every state of existential awareness, namely a position of seeing herself squashed and squeezed out of existence, at any meaningful level, and being pressurized to do so by friends, family and environment, becoming guilt-ridden and in danger of becoming isolated, mechanical and developing a depressive illness as a purely secondary phenomena. The business of homoeopathy is not just to prescribe the similimum remedy but also to be sensitive and aware to every aspect and depth of the patient, to plumb the depths so to speak, and to allow all levels to emerge and only then to prescribe. Once the level of disturbance is ascertained then a remedy and its potency can be correctly given.

Without adequate treatment, the danger of developing a physical illness, perhaps a rheumatoid arthritis state, or a skin condition like eczema or psoriasis, possibly a metabolic upset as diabetes, if there is a hereditary gene in the background to act as a pointer to which particular disease to develop. Other disturbing possibilities could be colitis, obesity, or more obvious psychological syndromes as anxiety-panic attacks or agoraphobia.

Note that anguish implies that the basic person in depth is under tension and compression with the external symptoms of anxiety, tension, irritability, panic, tears or insomnia as purely secondary and surface manifestations.

The Modalities for Existential Anguish

Better for absorption, involvement, dialogue, contact and acceptance. Worse for people who reassure, who make demands, for superficial chat, unexpected arrivals and hold-up generally as in a traffic queue or supermarket check-point (*Natrum mur.*).

The underlying feeling in anguish is one of non-attachment within the deepest self, like a bird without a nest or crag to rest on, or a ball, rattling around a billiard table, but where there is no pocket – really no position of security. They always feel vulnerable and at risk if they are themselves.

There is a reality in all of this and it is not delusional. People are intolerant, they don't understand, they do make pressures and demands. You do have to conform to be loved and accepted in the majority of Western societies.

A Comparison of Existential Anguish with Anxiety

Anxiety usually has an infantile root to it, a neurotic level of infantile-parental attachment with either ambivalence or idealization, in any case one of prolonged or excessive attachment. There may or may not be a desire to create or need a dialogue. Nearly always there are unresolved areas of earlier development, or a complete stoppage at an earlier stage with problems of suppressed jealousy, resentment, competition, rivalry, stimulating often greed and envy leading to destructive attitudes. Problems of identifying with a person who is also resented, often causes retaliatory fears and confusion. All of this creates a muddled picture of the identity, with weakness, uncertainty and lack of confidence.

Note that Kent gives the following black letter remedies for anguish and anxiety (Chapter 7) – *Aconitum*, *Belladonna*, *Arsenicum*, *Cannabis indica*, *Calcarea*, *Causticum*, *Digitalis*, *Hepar sulph.*, *Platina*. These are best prescribed 'high' whenever anguish is diagnosed.

22

Mood Swings

These are normal and natural for us all to some degree. The everyday pressures and vicissitudes of pressurized provocative living, the frustrations of reality external difficulties combined with the more subtle media-psychological pressures of commercial origin to be better or different, all add to instability or lack of confidence. Psychological uncertainty or confusion can easily develop in the susceptible and an abrupt change of mood stem from deeper internal doubts, pressures and impulses.

Such problems are always highlighted by the menstrual cycle or just before, when all feelings are more available, nearer the surface and are the reason at this time for the frequent show of tears or irritability.

Men tend to bottle-up much more, to contain and keep down for a variety of reasons, including the educational one. This is the main reason for the higher incidence in men than women of the civilization diseases, like duodenal ulcer, blood pressure and heart-disease.

Mood swings are normal given the intensity of present social changes and pressures affecting most of us where literally no one can be certain of a job or position five years from now. Where there is added temperamental instability from a variety of causes including hereditary or traumatic reasons, this is an additional factor and often accounts for irritability, short-fuse reactions and poor controls with a sudden 'down' into a trough of despair, futility and tears. Mood swings may be severe for some, with swings from one day to the next, the partner never sure from which side of the bed they will alight that morning, so that the pattern of life is one of unpredictability and uncertainty. Life varies from a 'high' of laughter, confidence, energy, achievement, celebration and 'joie de vivre' to pessimism, defeat and despair.

Remedies for Mood Swings

Apis – mainly for restless excitability with hysterical features of agitation and many *Pulsatilla* characteristics. More agitated than the latter, the swings are greater.

Arsenicum – Extreme, acute agitation, with insomnia, over-active mind, restless and irritable. Time passes slowly, causing impatience. Underlying lack of confidence.

Calcarea – For the constitutionally weak. Slow. A dreamer and low-achiever, often impatient and irritable and frequently a late developer in all areas.

Natrum mur. – Much less active than the two former remedies without the almost complete lethargy of *Calcarea*. Moodiness from tears to uncontrollable laughter, but basically a 'loner', irritable, with little confidence. Provoked by contact and company and any situation they are unable to control.

Nux vomica – The remedy for the 'stressed-out' businessman, unable to delegate, with a short-fuse, coming home tired and irritable, wakes up jaded and exhausted. He is full of complaints about the incompetence of others, and spills over with zealous moods of self-righteousness and rage.

Phosphorus – The female equivalent of *Nux vom.*, but more popular, artistic, sensitive and less arrogant, with more time for others and time to listen. Weak temperamentally, there are flashes of feeling – tears, depression and rage, needing others. Less zealous and confident than *Nux vom.*

Pulsatilla – Valuable for all types of changing variability of mood and temperament in the male or female. There is variation in everything, from one moment to another, even their depths of despair or the 'highs' of enthusiasm and optimism. All are short-lived and barely has one mood pattern or set of feelings been expressed when they are just as quickly erased by the least suggestion to the contrary. They are so unsure of themselves that all feelings are fleeting and temporary which makes for their enormous vulnerability.

Manic Depressive Illness

A much more severe, psychotic condition with severe alternating hypomanic mood disturbance and severe depression with suicidal intent. The mood disturbances contain the characteristic diagnostic feature of a break with reality and delusional features. A well-organized, plausible system of beliefs may be present with impressive features stated with conviction which given a convincing ring to it by the intermingling of present or past factual events and names. This gives the delusional fabric a convincing ring of truth and authenticity, perpetuating and reinforcing the delusions.

The patient is often middle-aged, male or female, with a marked excess of energy, exhausting to try and keep up with. Working or talking night and day, on the telephone, running up enormous bills, not containable or answerable to reason, they quickly become agitated, restless and aggressive. Laughing, full of stories, taking rash decisions when in a position of authority they may put both business and family security into complete jeopardy. At times they are close to a paranoid illness with delusions of global plots, the FBI, the Russians, industrial espionage or sinister plans involving the sinking of ships or the 'downing' of aeroplanes. They are nearly always 'in the know' with access to inside secret information and a prime target or vulnerable. Names are dropped impressively at every opportunity, with over-articulation, ceaseless toing and froing, without rest, proper meals or sleep.

This takes its toll physically so that they are at risk to becoming more ill with an acute physical condition such as a duodenal ulcer, a stroke from elevated blood pressure or a heart attack.

Physical complications are however rare and they seem to develop an immunity to such illnesses, which would be inevitable to anyone else with the same degree of over-activity. Intelligence and plausibility adds to the difficulty of making a diagnosis and because of the surfeit of energy and lack of insight, it is often impossible for them to see that they are ill or have a problem. The usual complaint is of other people's incompetence or that they are the victim of an international plot. They are often suspicious of doctors. A treatment order for compulsory admission may be required in some cases although it is best avoided if possible, because it tends to worsen the condition and increase the delusional certainty that doctors, friends and family are trying to have them committed, locked-up as mad in an asylum – to get rid of them. In general treatment and response to homoeopathy is encouraging.

Remedies for Manic Depression

Agaricus (Amanita toad stool) – An excellent remedy for extremes of mood with excitement and depression closely following each other. Note the characteristic twitching and poor circulation.

Anacardium orientale – Anger, irritability, vehement rage and swearing with loss of control, delusions, suicidal determined intentions.

Medorrhinum – For the more psychotic unreal states, often grandiose. Impatience is marked and everything is rushed and in a hurry. Better for sea air.

Platina – For the profoundly disturbed, arrogant states of superiority and ecstasy with visual and bodily disturbances of imagery, others seem smaller and far away. Close to a schizophrenic state of unreality and dissociation.

Lachesis – For the more aggressive, dangerous, homicidal, paranoidal secretive states of delusional conviction and certainty. Jealousy and suspicion are always marked.

Aconitum – For sudden acute traumatic cases, of recent onset with an acute situation of fear or shock, sometimes following the sudden loss of limb as in an industrial accident. Excitability and delusional certainty are marked.

Belladonna – For hypomanic phases of violence and restlessness, difficult to control and sensitive to the least approach, touch, jar or draught.

23

Psychosomatic Illness

The common problem of ill-health where there is a powerful underlying emotional causative factor being funnelled through a physical pathway of indirect outlet and expression causing a variety of symptoms – some benign and relatively insignificant, others more dangerous – sometimes even to life itself.

It is difficult to distinguish a truly psychosomatic condition from the 'completely' physical condition because in nearly every physical illness, without exception there is an emotional factor which prepares the ground for illness – alters the physiological terrain or soil, changes the healthy position of physiological homoeostasis and balance to one of dis-ease and imbalance. When this happens, the essential defences of vital energy are weakened or lost and former 'friends' and symbiotic neighbours can become hostile invaders.

Psychosomatic illness implies however something more than an emotional string or causative factors – it suggests a much more powerful emotional force or drive that is not being channelled through the proper psychological expressive cathartic channels of emotional release and 'outburst'. Usually a dialogue of expression and understanding release has not occurred or prevented tensions rising to unbearable limits. It is often these feelings which are given a physical exit and which makes them much more slow to respond to conventional remedies – including a well-indicated homoeopathic prescription. You may argue that this happens anyway, and that psychosomatic is just a question of degree and intensity. I sympathize with this view but here it is also very much a question of degree and the intensity of emotional discharge via the physical pathways.

In nearly every case, the individual concerned is of 'sensitive' make-up, usually non-aggressive, weakly assertive, and intellectual with a natural artistic-sensitive side. Aggressive-competitive sports and activity outlets are often limited – often present in the *Lycopodium* or *Pulsatilla* temperament and constitutional picture.

Symptoms may be reversed, controlled or eradicated by hypnosis – even made to appear. The TB Mantoux-test reaction can be eradicated on one side which raises the problem of where allergy fits into the psychosomatic spectrum, especially something so obviously physical as sensitivity to the protein of the Mantoux injection and seemingly psychologically uncomplicated. The importance of stress and psychological factors in a TB vaccination programme comes into question here, especially where a Mantoux is negative or vaguely positive or unclear. If you have no Mantoux reaction – supposedly you have no immunity and only the positive cutaneous allergic response is indicative of previous infection and immunity. The indication for BCG vaccination against TB rests on a negative reaction, but it seems possible that undue stress may give false, negative responses to a condition where immunity already exists or the opposite.

In psychosomatic disease, there is nearly always a family history of the same disease in one member of the family – often a parent or grandparent, which provides the hereditary strand in the aetiology, in addition to the psychological one already mentioned.

Major psychosomatic illnesses usually include the following: asthma, colitis, eczema, hay-fever, the allergic summer problems of catarrh or sinusitis, migraine, blood-pressure, peptic ulcer, gall-bladder disease, obesity. Heart attack is usually considered to be a disease of civilization, a stress illness with a major underlying psychological cause. They may also be grouped closely to the psychosomatic conditions if not included in them.

The problem does not seem to be environmental, as much as an increase of susceptibility to the environmental irritants. It is as common to see identical twins in the surgery – one with a psychosomatic problem and the other quite different from any related or psychosomatic symptoms. In my practice I have identical twin boys aged 8 who always come together with the mother. One twin has severe asthma since infancy, apparently related to pollen although in more recent years the problem has been present throughout the year with numerous bouts of hospitalization, steroid treatments and oxygen tents. The other twin is quite symptom-free. My patient is smaller and less well-built than his brother, but this may be a purely secondary outcome of the chest problem. He is purely catching up with the home treatments. More anxious, clinging and of sensitive-dependent psychological make-up, he clings to his mother earfully, crying or whimpering whenever I listen to his chest. But this too may be the secondary outcome of the numerous admissions in the past and fear of doctors and further hospitalization. Since homoeopathic treatment with *Phosphorus*, *Medorrhinum* and *Luna* – all symptoms are worse for the new moon, also *Timothy grass pollen* the symptoms have lessened and he has put on weight, but the problem is still there from time to time and remains a worry for the family because of the danger to life of the asthmatic spasm when severe and uncontrollable.

In many cases, desensitization has been specifically carried out using a variety of allergens and proteins, including eggs, chocolate, dog, cat or horse hair, and house dust or mites. Often the effects are not satisfactory or lasting and I rarely use them. A specific allergic factor should always be excluded when it can be found but in my experience this is rare and in most cases there are few specific allergens to be found and the cause has to be labelled non-specific.

Both asthma and colitis can become extremely dangerous illnesses and not uncommonly the acute illness follows within a few weeks, a stressful situation where for a variety of reasons, including temperament and 'expediency', a show of anger and feeling was not allowed expression or outlet. Indignation at the situation is usually suppressed. (Note the importance and value of *Staphisagria* here.)

All psychosomatic problems give a positive reaction to homoeopathy. Only in the young child with asthma or ulcerative colitis where there is danger to life in a crisis, is admission to hospital or a special unit required so that often essential conventional treatments can be given because the homoeopathic one cannot 'hold' the situation or the crisis has occurred between appointments and the doctor is not available. In such states of emergency, where resistance and vital energy is low, homoeopathy takes a secondary supportive position to the conventional approach. I often give the parents of my young asthmatic patients an 'emergency pack', usually in high potency of the known remedy for such an emergency so that they have something in reserve, and can cope better and treat any severe spasm as early as possible. This gives confidence to the mother as is reflected in their handling of a susceptible child. But such measures do not always work. You may argue that such measures do not always work. You may argue that such measures only anticipate a situation and may indeed suggest it to the mind of the susceptible patient or parent. Perhaps it is better to let the attacks actually occur, rather than to anticipate them, although the 'emergency pack' gives more confidence, reassurance and relaxation. Homoeopathy is often used as a prophylactic, quite properly and in keeping with the best traditions. But in the final analysis it is the patient that matters most and not theory or traditions. On the whole I am in favour of a 'standby' for anxious parents with a weak, susceptible and at-risk child. The whole problem of prophylaxis and whether to prescribe in anticipation needs to be assessed for each individual child and family and the availability of the doctor concerned.

Many parents are able prescribers themselves and well able to help a child in an emergency – often only needing a minimum of support and advice. Others are different and panic or worsen a situation because they project their own fears and inadequacy into it.

In general and without going into specifics, which is not the point of this chapter, it is best to give the constitutional prescription wherever possible in the highest potency available and in a very severe condition to repeat it hourly until there is an improvement. I often follow this by a specific allergen remedy, where this is known or of proved value – usually in the 6th centesimal or 3X potency three to four times daily.

Case History – Allergic Urticaria due to Brown-tail Moth (Euproctis Chysorrhoea)

The patient was a university student aged 20, working for a research degree. He came with a specific allergic sensitivity rash to the Brown-tail moth which he was researching. He developed a severe skin reaction from the least contact with the caterpillar severely limiting his ability to work in the field. The main symptoms were of itchy redness and raised white wheals as is typical of urticaria. The Brown-tail moth is important on two accounts – the extent of its defoliating habits in caterpillar form and its link with Epidemic Urticaria. In Shanghai in 1972 over half a million people were involved with Epidemic Urticaria needing medical attention, a quarter of the population of the city. Severe outbreaks have also occurred in the Netherlands (1980), Yugoslavia, Poland and on the Black Sea coast. In England it has caused severe problems on the south coast of Sussex and along the Thames estuary. The eggs are laid in July and August and after five months of hibernation, the young lava emerge and devastate the leaves of the host plants, especially the Oak, Poplar, Lime, Plane and Forsythia. Several moultings of lava skin occur before they finally reach maturity as the fully grown caterpillar in June.

The problem is the barbed, missile-shaped hair of the caterpillar which contains backward-pointed irritant barbs which can penetrate the skin, mucous membrane or conjunctiva by handling, contact, inhalation or indirect contact. The toxic, irritant barbs are found in the air or sometimes several miles from the actual vicinity of the caterpillar's main site of defoliation. Each barb contains a toxin at its point which has not yet been identified but is of histamine type and a protein compound of high molecular weight.

Although the problem is usually a localized one with painful itching and urticaria with redness and swelling, in two cases death in the UK from asthma was provoked by an attack directly due to the caterpillar hairs. Sufferers from hay-fever, asthma and eczema are aggravated by the barbs with an unusually severe reaction. Blair reports two cases of blindness (permanent) and others where urticarial eruptions lasted for several months.

My patient provided me with moulting samples of the caterpillar, which when handled caused him a marked urticarial reaction within 20 minutes. These moulting samples were made up into a 6th centesimal potency by the Hahnemann method. While they were in preparation, he was given *Urtica* in the 10M potency also *Rhus tox.* in the 6C potency to be taken daily if *Urtica* failed to give relief. He was 70% improved within 48 hours by homoeopathic *Urtica* to the incredulity of every member of the university department and able to continue his work and research again with only minimal discomfort. Use of the specific moulting sample in potency completely cured the condition in a period of weeks.

24

Depression

I have already dealt with the more general forms of infantile and adult depression and depression of the elderly. I would like to deal here with some of the other more specific types of depression also seen in practice.

Puerperal Depression

A 'low' commonly occurs after childbirth in most women, from a combination of fatigue, anticipatory anxiety about the actual delivery and the health of the child, insomnia, frustration to some degree, and the demanding, often routine tie of suddenly becoming a mother. In true puerperal depression, there is more than just irritability, frustration and sometimes resentment. A most overwhelming depression occurs, with psychotic element present and entering into both mood and thought processes, distorting reality. This leads to delusional formation, especially of being bad, ugly, unloved and unloving, inadequate. She feels different from the other mothers because she has been singled out, is controlled, interfered with, talked about over the radio, poisoned or has a

188

special mission. There may be homicidal phantasies or compulsions towards the baby – 'put into the mind', or that the child is not hers, has been changed or interfered with. She sometimes feels full of guilt or that she 'has sinned' – as part of the delusional guilt and depression.

Remedies for Puerperal Depression

Consider the following remedies, using high potencies wherever possible.

Sepia – Where there is a combination of negative indifference towards the child, and frightening overwhelming rejecting or destructive phantasies.

Platina – Where irritable resentment and indignation combines with a distorted, enlarged body image and phantasies of delusional importance or greatness.

Nat. mur. – Tears, inadequacy, exhaustion, cannot cope with the baby, but less deluded.

Arnica – Where the condition follows a prolonged, drawn-out exhausting confinement.

Aconitum – Fear is the predominant emotion, delusional in intensity and restlessness and absolute certainty as to the intentions of others to destroy her.

Ignatia – Psychosis follows a sudden loss as with a stillborn, grief or shock.

Staphisagria – Irritable hostility with resentment, indignation and revenge marked, especially where the birth has been drawn-out, painful or surgical (forceps).

Cimicifuga, Actea Racemisa (Black Snake Root) – The illness follows a severe delusional course with confusion. Hallucinations are marked. The illness may follow a fairly chronic course usually over weeks or months but once resolved it does not usually recur unless there is another confinement when it may occur again after the delivery – sometimes in a second and third pregnancy, but always during the puerperium. In other cases it only occurs on the one occasion and there is no further recurrence in subsequent deliveries.

Agitated Depression

Common in the elderly but also common in the adult, there is a chronic long-standing condition, present for months, even years. Masochism is a feature, often with a long-suffering spouse or relative who bears the brunt of the barely concealed sadism of the patient which is rarely absent in one form or other. Groaning, complaining that nothing helps, or is any good, that no medicine, and no doctor, is useful and that everyone fails. Nothing pleases, and nothing works; he or she feels lost, finished, doomed and dying. The masochism and self-centredness is associated with bizarre, frequently localized head or body pains, constant and agonizing which nothing seems to relieve. Insomnia and preoccupation with chronic constipation due partly to lack of exercise, an irregular diet and endless laxatives, completes the picture. Delusional beliefs of a localized nature may be present. They cannot rest by day or night, and are up and down, here and there, driving both themselves and their family to the limits of patience, kindness and tolerant understanding. 'Would try a saint' – is close to the mark, and often they have found one in their partner who has devoted their lives uncomplainingly to them and in consequence has only rarely reached their full potential and identity.

190

Remedies for Agitated Depression

The following remedies act on combination of depression and agitation and should be considered. *Zincum met.*, *Nat. mur.*, *Belladonna*, *Rhus tox.*, *Mag. carb.*, *Naja*, *Nitric ac.*

Psychotic Depression

This closely resembles puerperal depression but is not provoked by childbirth. It can occur at any age, with a frank schizophrenia or schizophrenic type of illness. The previous personality has often been somewhat bizarre, untidy, withdrawn and schizoid (*Sulphur*). In others, the previous personality was essentially 'normal' – but too much so, with marked insecurity, control, and obsessional tendencies. The major psychological problem is a fragmenting of personality leading to severe delusional state, which undermine relationships and healthy functioning, by projection of personality-fragments into others and other situations. Such fragments always 'boomerang' back at the person, however extensive the personality break-up. Even in a psychosis you can't get away from yourself, however far you travel, and here the journey is as far away as possible from self by flight and elusion into another imaginary world. The outer experience is felt to be so flimsy, vague and uncertain, that life and contacts become a matter of guesswork, supposition and conjecture. At other times things seem absolutely concrete and certain. Fears are marked, usually persecutory, also hallucinations and depression which frequently borders onto a suicidal frame of mine and preoccupation.

Remedies for Psychotic Depression

Stramonium – Where excitement and restlessness is marked with hallucinations.

Hyoscyamus – More intensely agitated and violent, with hallucinations, mania, difficult to control or reassure. Intolerant of any form of covering.

Belladonna – For less violent reactions, with restless delusional behaviour but not so destructive. Heat is a feature.

Tarantula hisp. – Recommended for the most violent and destructive behaviour. Like *Sepia* it is also better for quick movements such as dancing and music soothes.

Lachesis – For the more suspicious, paranoid illness.

Sulphur – Where there is more of a frank schizophrenic illness without undue restless violence and agitation. The whole inner world dominates the picture of reality and there is a tendency to idealize their own imagery so that the least unattractive external object can become the subject of endless ecstasy.

Suicidal Depression

There is despair, hopelessness and a determination to end life. Failure, desperation, fear are all characteristic of the more severe and black depressive moods, often acutely so, but frequently the problem that has recurred over a period of years and suicide has been thought about during 'low' times since adolescence. Often nothing has been 'done' about it because of the family or simply not knowing how. It can occur from childhood onwards, is very common in late adolescence – the university

192

tudent, pressured by tutor, family and self alike, o make life a nightmare and a burden, with failure nthinkable and intolerable. Increasingly in the ame age group, is the out-of-work youth with no rospects of meaningful employment in the foreseeable future. It is also common in adults as well as he elderly. Sometimes suicide becomes part of a eliberate and conscious decision, a pact even between the couple – to end life at a certain age or ate before the anticipated problems of deterioraion and dependency occur as an unthinkable cross o bear. For them the solution is to prevent the roblems of old age from happening and to deterninedly 'have out' before they happen. The devasating effect on the children and grandchildren is ot considered at the time or denied, but is a ointer to the intensely selfish features of the suicial act.

Remedies of Suicidal Depression

Aurum met. – The person cannot be roused by any neans from their depression and there is a determination to end life as soon as possible. Cardiac ymptoms are often associated.

Natrum sulph. – The depression is of an endogenous type, with early morning waking, silent depresion, withdrawal and determination to suicide. Chest problems are common.

Nux vomica – There is a most irritable illumoured intolerant spasmodic depression with udden, dangerous impulses to violent suicide, ften as successful as they are determined.

Argentum nit. – For the more obsessional, compulive type of problem, with impulses to throw themelves from a high window, a bridge or into water.

Not often acted upon, but this sometimes occurs a way out of their intolerable scruples.

Alumina – For milder forms, less impulsive b ruminated upon over the years. There is an obse sional fear of knives or any potential instrument suicide. Constipated.

China – Suicidal impulses from exhaustion; wor out, hopeless, nothing to live for. Particularly value for suicidal depression of the elderly.

Veratrum alb. – The problem here is more of psychosis, with mute sullen withdrawal and ofte determined a well-planned suicidal determinatior

Ignatia – For suicidal depression during an acu period of grief and mourning.

Hysterical Depression

The danger of hysterical depression is always that cry for help – a suicidal threat or gesture will g wrong and end in needless tragedy. This has hap pened many times over the years in depressive ac that could have been anticipated and preventec but they were not taken seriously at the time. A with all hysterical manifestations, there is the typ cal combination of insecurity, attention-seekin behaviour, immaturity and variability of mooc easily lifted by praise or reassurance and just a quickly touched-off again by a seemingly critica remark or misunderstood turn of phrase. There an irritable loneliness – because they rarely give out enough of themselves to establish a carin relationship and are too self-orientated and self absorbed. Often there has been a chain of 'wrong inappropriate relationships, always ending badl over the years, and always the fault of the othe person – who has not given or understood then enough. A dependent attachment to one or both parents is usually a problem that has never been fully resolved and accounts for much of their infantile attitudes and immaturity.

Remedies for Hysterical Depression

Ignatia – One of the best remedies, with a variety of psychosomatic complaints and often an old problem of an unresolved loss or separation.

Pulsatilla – Must be considered in all cases where there is a passive manipulating temperament. Tearfulness and intolerance of heat is typical, with variability in all things, even from moment to moment during a bout of severe depression.

Cimicifuga racemosa – Sudden unpredictable or impulsive hysterical behaviour including suicidal threats and gestures.

Asafoetida – Especially where fainting and collapse are marked.

Moschus – Useful in the adolescent with immaturity, no confidence and a variety of fears and convictions of an obsessional nature, especially of disease or dying.

Valerian – For the more severe, 'malignant' hysterical condition, bordering on the psychotic, with a variety of disturbed imagery and always worse in the evenings.

25

Fears and Phobias

Agoraphobia

Fear of exposed, open places is the commonest of the phobias and is usually but not invariably a female condition. The problem can arise at any age, more especially in the 30–50 age group. In the child it can occur when there is fear of leaving the mother and security of the home, often with associated truancy problems and an ambivalent attitude towards the mother. In the young, agoraphobia frequently manifests, with boys or girls, as a school phobia. It may also occur in the elderly of either sex as part of a senile state of delusion or confusion.

The origin of the condition is often obscure. In one patient aged 55 agoraphobia followed a period of grief after the sudden loss of her husband through a heart attack some four years previously. Since then she had felt constantly vulnerable, panicky and terrified of collapse and dying which worsened at the anniversary date of his loss. She felt anxious, weak and fearful (*Aconitum*).

This patient had the classic fear of traffic, in her case linked with a near-fatal road accident that occurred before the heart attack when her husband was driving. Moving fast into a motorway from a slip road, one side of the car was ripped off. Her husband climbed out of the car unhurt but nevertheless at the time the wife was convinced he was fatally injured.

This same fear was revitalized after his actual death and is still associated with driving and traffic of any degree. The whole phobia has strong links with mourning. Any talk of her husband still leads to tears, sadness, a sense of loss revealing an unresolved psychological situation (*Ignatia*, *Pulsatilla*).

Prior to her bereavement there had been no previous psychiatric history or similar symptoms and she had held a responsible senior position without any sense of inadequacy or insecurity – perhaps always shouldering other people's problems and never admitting or expressing her own vulnerability. If anything, there was an over-close, dependent, exclusive marital relationship.

This patient's agoraphobia contained the typical boundary' situation of a boxed area, well-defined, where she can safely drive and walk without panic or anxiety and with a major busy road as a boundary on one side of the box. She can cross outside this barrier only on a quiet Sunday morning and then with great anxiety. The least delay, blockage or anticipated hold-up causes fear, panic and dread of not getting back to the safety of home.

Her insecurity is given an outside representation: a wide road or a busy one is the site of potential panic and fear. There is always a lot of aggression associated with these problems. Snappy anger, fear of violence and loss of control are never far away – often emerging as frustration at delay or

197

where there is a sudden demand for conversation
An unexpected visitor has to be coped with
Although a relief as well as an unwelcome threat, i
is only with a major effort that social niceties are
adhered to and politeness is almost a tour de force
The underlying violence makes for more poignan
feelings of loss of control and adds to the problem
either of going out or fears of going to pieces and
madness.

Major Remedies

Aconitum – Where fear of dying and collapse are a
certainty and indeed predicted, also where acute
fear has been the prime stimulus to the phobic
condition.

Arnica – Where the onset followed shock o
trauma.

Arsenicum – Where restless agitation, weaknes:
and phobic anxiety are predominant.

Aurum met. – Depression with palpitations and
hypersensitivity to traffic noise or smells.

Nat. mur. – Phobia in the nervous loner, with a
dislike of people, contact, noise or disturbance o
the daily routine.

Platina – Pride and aggression are marked with
arrogance and enormous lack of confidence under
the surface and only just barely hidden, which
makes for vulnerability.

Claustrophobia

This is the opposite condition to agoraphobia with
a fear of being trapped, shut-in, crushed, unable to
get out or escape. Sufferers hate any crowded, busy
situation. They need a bolt-hole for every social

occasion, especially at a concert, theatre or cinema. There is a feeling of being closeted and choked, of needing fresh air; even a fear of collapsing and dying. A hot, stuffy atmosphere has adverse physical or psychological effects (*Pulsatilla*).

All too often, this phobia is a reflection of inner over-control of which the person may be unaware. For instance, fear of being in a lift or cupboard symbolizes denial of the sufferer's true feelings and impulses about another situation – an unhappy marriage or family problems they are unwilling to admit. Sometimes, although this is rare, the condition may have arisen as a result of being locked in a dark cupboard in childhood as a means of punishment.

For the majority, claustrophobia reflects their inner world. They keep themselves – all impulses and feelings – shut in and tightly closeted away for safety, in case they come out uncontrollably and with too much force after many years of denial. There is usually a strongly ambivalent attitude towards a marital or family situation.

The unconscious wish is to opt out. But for a variety of reasons, either real or temperamental, this is not possible. What is really feared is more an aggressive outburst or break-out rather than of being shut-in. In most cases, passivity and non-aggression are the order of the day, control of self and others being typical.

Major Remedies

Arg. nit. – The most important remedy with fear of any enclosed situation, especially one with heat. Fear of being trapped. Fear of diarrhoea in a public situation.

Carbo veg. – Weakness and collapse, aggravated by imposed contact with others. Sweating and panic and near-collapse. Gastric symptoms marked with flatulence.

Pulsatilla – Vulnerability, weakness, tearfulness, passivity, worse for a public, stuffy situation. Faintness. Can't get breath.

Sulphur – Confusion and control of boundaries with an unreal phantasy type of existence.

Eating in Public

Sufferers experience inappropriate anxiety, panic or fear in any situation on which the hands or mouth are involved and on display, either when handling food and drink or eating when others are near or felt to be in the vicinity watching and judging them.

In many ways this is an infantile position, demonstrating a failure to grow and progress beyond the early oral stage of infantile development and the need to be observed. The natural course of development is delayed, therefore, and this to some extent affects the whole of life – relationships, work and sexuality. Such people express themselves predominantly through the mouth area only. This does not usually undermine adult dialogue and meaningful conversation which has a later level of development.

There is over-evaluation of eating, table manners and food. They are typically fussy and faddy about what they like and will eat and what will upset them, picking at their food and taking only small amounts. Often they seem to be re-creating earlier experiences and sometimes traumas, particularly of actually having been force-fed by an over-anxious mother or grandmother.

The oral area is one of major exhibitionism and the ever-present fear is an unconscious wish to bite, suck and take in too greedily. Fears of fainting, collapse and dying are common. Indeed, anything that may make an obvious show and a drama is both feared and unconsciously wished for and sought.

They are the most messy, clumsy eaters at all times, tipping or spilling something over themselves or, more often, others near them and generally being a nuisance. They tend to be far too intense emotionally in a childlike, obvious way. The combination of food and the public situation acts as an overwhelmingly powerful stimulus and signal to make a 'show' – and often a mess too. Hence the fear and the anxiety at one and the same time.

Recommended Remedies

Lycopodium – Typically clumsy, ill-at-ease in a social situation where the mouth and gastric functioning is concerned. Worriers who anticipate disaster. Accident-prone and infantile behind a thin veil of social aplomb.

Gelsemium – Irritable and wants to be left alone. They feel everyone is looking at them. There are strong feelings of anxiety in public places and weakness and collapse and fainting.

Medorrhinum – Typical dread of public places. Time passes too slowly and the meal and the evening seem interminably drawn out, causing fidgety restlessness. Fear of being trapped and dying, only better outside and by the seaside, eating on the terrace.

Plumbum – Fear of a hypochondriacal nature of

being poisoned or ill when eating. Will never ea
mushrooms or anything 'chancy' in a restaurant
Very sensitive digestive systems. Severe and absolute constipation at times, often with attacks o
colic.

Phosphoric Acid – Weakness and collapse with
fear and panic are the main problem. Going out
and meeting people are dreaded, with the certainty
of collapse or fainting. Totally lacking energy.

Silicea – Timid dread of meeting a new situation.
Clumsy, weak and awkward. Panicky and no
confidence in themselves, often from lack of social
experience over the years.

The Opposite Sex

Here there is far too much primitive, infantile
emotion poured into later genital levels of expression and psychological development, drowning
them with early needs, feelings and priorities. The
genital level fails to develop properly and with
well-defined boundaries to keep out overwhelming
earlier tendencies. Sufferers cannot develop
mature, sharing, loving adult relationships.

All this makes for a sexuality that is a threat
because it is distorted, overwhelmed and made
frightening by earlier imagery which should have
been more fully integrated into the whole by being
left behind or only allowed expression in a more
controlled way – perhaps expressed as part of the
infinite variety in fore- and love-play, but not
overshadowing all else. Especially important is the
basic sharing, trust and giving of the self.

The most common basic fear is of sexual inadequacy, rejection, laughter, failure, blushing, self-
consciousness, not being loved and, sometimes, of

not responding and loving, of being felt unworthy. It is an extremely painful and lonely, immature position – natural for many in early adolescence. Unless there has been a trauma to fixate a block at this age and level, it is usually overcome quite naturally by being outgrown and is not a major problem.

With excessive anxiety, the whole genital and sexual situation has become distorted by phantasy, made grotesque, unreal. At times it may trickle over into adult perversion as a means of attempting some sort of release and orgasm, but rarely does a relationship develop unless dialogue and acceptance with some giving and sharing can be achieved.

Homoeopathy may need to be combined here with psychotherapy in the sense of more regular and close meetings for a time, with the homoeopathic remedy facilitating the whole process of release, confidence, change and maturation. Naturally these meetings can be spaced out with improvement from weekly to fortnightly and then monthly as the patient's confidence builds up.

Major Remedies

Pulsatilla – The person is always unsure of themselves and insecure, lacking confidence and maturity, especially in a sexual situation. Passivity and timidity are marked at all times except in close, familiar situation when they can bully. Display is a powerful part of the make-up, often hysterical in type.

Ignatia – Loss of confidence since break-up of a previous relationship with a sense of hurt, panic and fear and often grief and loss, hankering after the past because of fear of the present.

Calcarea – Weakness, shyness, inexperience, immaturity. Confidence is not their strong point in any situation. The basic personality is often deeply disturbed and based much more on phantasy rather than experience, maturity and previous involvements.

Appropriate Remedy

Experienced users of homoeopathy will find helpful Dr Trevor Smith's guide to remedies effective in coping with fears and phobias. Use a 30c potency. Anyone new to homoeopathy, or inexperienced, who is suffering from the symptoms described, should consult a homoeopath who will prescribe the most appropriate remedy and potency.

26

Hysteria

In many ways hysteria is opposite to anguish, and the most superficial of the psychological states. It is also the most ego-centric and perhaps the most vulnerable because it lacks depth. The whole of the adult personality is rooted in the infantile, still at that level and has never really managed to progress far from it – hence the often enviable youthful appearance, or childish physical impression sometimes to the point of being grotesque or 'mutton dressed as lamb'. In every case eternal youth is sought and courted, and the strength of the cosmetic industry and beauty salon is often largely due to their support.

The overwhelming problem is how to stay eternally beautiful and youthful in order to please – ultimately the parents, but if they are no longer alive or in an immediate relationship, the same pattern applies. In order to be accepted and loved, there is the conviction that it is the young and the beautiful who are loved and wanted. There is infantile attachment to one or both parents, often ambivalently, at times vehemently negative, or the tie is one of idealization and strongly positive feelings. The whole parental link may be rationalized on the grounds of illness or the need for dependency, but it is the infantile attitude, to the exclusion of all else, which gives the diagnosis.

Jealousy and competition are marked because of endless comparisons with any other person who is seen as a threat or rival for the love, attention and affection – of which they feel starved and must have in order to survive. But there is little real love because it is the capacity to demand and to take that is strong, rather than their ability to give out or to enfold.

There is typical childish need for attention-seeking reassurance, which is constant and never more than temporarily satisfied. This is combined with an often embarrassing necessity to be always in the limelight with a kind of provocative, dancing behaviour – feeling and acting as a child, and a collection of physical symptoms which have unconscious meaning, frequently of a sexual nature. Preoccupation with their self-orientated, narcissistic aims is to reassure against the dread of loss of love.

People, friends, and situations are 'collected' as purveyors of self-esteem and reassurance in the hopeless task of obtaining external proof of internal feelings of inadequacy or failure, worthlessness or loss. Much of this is because of their inability to give out sufficiently strong feelings of love and caring, weakened by fear or narcissism. Others are often seen as empty, not caring for them, largely because they themselves have not given out enough throughout their lives. This is also the reason for their dislike of others – often after the briefest encounter. The narcissism, is not so much self-love, but a demand for endless reassurance and being lovable.

There is an unachievable ideal of a love relationship which always eludes them, because they lack real interest or concern for others, always wanting a parental figure, and never failing to give out a stream of demands for attention. There is no insight into why they lack a meaningful relationship and a constant stream of admirers must be found or be courted, in order to reassure and to love them. This lessens depression and a sense of lonely inadequacy.

Where hysterical demands or 'needs' are channelled through physical channels they may develop bizarre, 'incurable' states of weakness or paralysis. All the symptoms have a powerful manipulative value and are worse when others are present, used to further reinforce their needs for sympathy and reassurance.

Because of emotional non-attachment, they feel un-attached physically, with a kind of weightless unreality, floating, planing, but never fully involved or themselves in any situation (*Nat. mur.*). This gives an impression of always surveying the scene, of looking down on life, as if from a tethered balloon, reflecting a dissociated, uninvolved part of them. The preoccupation with infantile phantasies, fears and needs, leave only a minor part of the adult self available for involvement, caring, and identification.

Recommended Remedies for Hysterical States and Unreality

Argentum nit. – Where fear and phobic elements predominate. Always worse for the presence of others, and for heat.

Asofoetida – Fainting is common in a public or

emotional situation when they feel the object of attention. Fear of fainting causes anxiety.

Belladonna – For hysterical fear, agitation, excitement, sometimes uncontrollable.

Calcarea – Weakness with chilly collapse, and obsessional features. Hypochondriasis and self-orientated. Irritable and manipulative.

Coffea – When agitation, tension, mood-changes are marked with insomnia, in spite of fatigue and exhaustion.

Gelsemium – Paralysing exhaustion or hysterical conversion paralysis of a limb or vocal chord. Tremor with fear and general lack of confidence.

Hyoscyamus – For the more malignant, near-psychotic form of hysteria with over-excitement, poor controls and potentially dangerous, self-destructive impulses. Always worse for lying down and at night.

Ignatia – Fear, with the typical hysterical contradictions and opposites. Changeable in mood and uncertain. Unpredictable and different in every symptom and conforming to no known pattern.

Kali carb. – For hysterical weakness, depression, over-anxious and dependent. Unable to tolerate being alone. Psychosomatic problems are associated, especially asthma or hay-fever. Conversion symptoms; weakness of one arm or leg, especially left-sided weakness.

Moschus – For the most dramatic, attention-seeking behaviour. Lump in throat.

Platina – Where the disturbance is of a more arrogant type and aggressive. There is isolation with few friends because of the spite and elevated sense of self-importance. Jealousy or suspicion may be a feature when bordering on a psychotic state.

Pulsatilla – Where changeable moods, tears, sympathy and depression are a feature. The mood changes from elation to tears, better for contact with others and for consolation. Sexual relationships are immature and often a major problem and preoccupation.

Valerian – Important where the problem is a severely dissociated state of mind with unreality, conversion symptoms and confusion.

Obsessional States and Hypochondriasis

An obsessional tendency in everyone to some extent, common as a superstitious need to 'touch wood', avoidance of ladders, spilling salt or breaking a mirror. These fears are very general and present in most countries and cultures. Like the superstitious act, the obsessional gesture is made to ward off an expected or imminent catastrophe – provoked by 'error', the Gods of Wrath waiting to inflict a true and just but usually terrifying punishment. Such thinking is a continuation of infantile attitudes and omnipotent thinking, with scruples and a variety of magical and rigid gestures or mannerisms as a kind of penance or appeasement to placate powerful (parental) punishing figures. Repeated acts and formulae are exacted from the self by a set of formulae and patterns, as a defence against the uncontrollable uncertainties of life, of fate and destiny.

To the obsessional mind, certainties are intolerable, even those of fate and they want guarantees, certainties, and absolutes for their own security, usually weakened by a combination of temperament, family influences, or trauma. According to Freudian theory, they are fixated at an early stage of personality development with over-emphasis on cleanliness, order and control. Metaphorically, not wanting to be caught with 'their pants down' which is their greatest fear, it gives a clue to toilet-training links. Freud recorded the principal character as pedantic, parsimonious and petulant attitudes.

Such control and arrangement is seen in the over-neat child with their toys, each neatly laid out in lines, or the game of not stepping on a pavement crack. In the adult it may take the form of being over-cautious, or double-checking and controlling in every area, living a carefully regulated life, but always fearing that something has been overlooked and will catch up, or find them off-guard.

The obsessional leads a narrow but regular ordered predictable life in everything, living by the clock, equally controlling anyone they are involved with. Their personal lives are as restricted as everything else about them.

Hypochondriasis is where depressive obsessional fears have crystallized upon a specific organ area especially the bowels. These become a preoccupation throughout life, especially such common problems as piles or body odour. The whole of life may be centred around keeping regular, trying yet another laxative or haemorrhoidal cream, another patent medicine, with no hope of recovery because their attitudes generally, lack of exercise and unbalanced diet reinforces to stasis, retention, and withholding. The physical problems and preoccupations are a reflection of mental constipation, but differ from hysterical symptoms, as less obviously infantile and manipulative in character.

Recommended Remedies for Obsessional States and Hypochondriasis

Arum met. – For a more depressive suicidal obsession, and the preoccupation with death or dying, melancholia and self-denigration.

Aconitum – Fears dominate everything in an obsessional way, ruminating on the certainty and conviction of their imminent death and incurable condition.

Anacardium – For more bizarre, inappropriate convictions and ideas which obsessionally turn round and around in the mind.

Hyoscyamus – For delusional fears and obsessional convictions, where suspicion and mistrust is a feature. Especially fear of water, bridges and drowning.

Cicuta – For a more paranoid obsessional state, silent, withdrawn and suspicious.

Cuprum met. – The remedy for spasm, both mentally as well as physically and sudden overactive obsessional states of doubting and dis-ease.

Ignatia – Hysterical states with obsessional features, especially after grief and loss.

Lachesis – Indicated where jealousy, suspicion or inadequacy is marked with an obsessional certainty that the partner is unfaithful. Depression borders on a paranoid-like state.

Stramonium – Where more hypo-manic features manifest as excitable, obsessional with little control and violent episodes, which are potentially dangerous. Often the mental states border on a psychotic condition.

Silicea – For more long-standing cases, where weakness and exhaustion are marked. Thin, undersized, both physically and mentally, they have no confidence. Avoidance of others adds to the inexperience and fears.

Pulsatilla – The remedy for variable states of mixed hysterical-obsessional illness, with rigid, fixed thinking and conviction. Constantly changeable, too passive and agreeable, unless sure of their ground, when they can be quite nasty or bullying. All symptoms are worse for heat.

Thuja – For more bizarre, obsessional states of hypochondriasis, especially of the elderly. The body is felt as rotting, brittle, made of glass, penetrated by a single nail or containing a live animal.

Veratrum alb. – Indicated for obsessional-depressive states of the puerperium, which may proceed to a frank psychotic condition.

Sulphur – Indicated for chronic insecurity problems, with obsessional defences and rather rigid controlled tendencies. The thought processes are vague and with *Sulphur* 'anything goes'. There may be a more disturbed centre to the illness, with marked uncertainty and the accumulation of splinters or fragments of ideas organized into a bizarre defence with scruples. The overall untidiness of mind and body, the grandiose phantasies with intolerance of heat is characteristic.

27

Grief and Loss

can be confidently affirmed that grief and loss
re part of everyone's experience from birth and
nfancy onwards and that growth and maturity are
mpossible without a break in some way from the
ast – the relinquishing of a cherished belief, con-
iction or position in favour of another. As we pass
hrough life so too we pass through a whole chain
f significant experiences, some more meaningful
han others. Some are apparently small at the time,
vhilst others are massive experiences which entail
 giving-up, an abandoning and therefore a loss.
All of these – the apparently insignificant as well as
he 'events' – mark us in some way and leave their
race or scars. From the cradle, the cot, the breast
r bottle, through weaning and on to school, grow-
ng up, maturing implies the giving up of a
avoured position of security.

We grow, experience and mature at the cost of
xposing ourselves to new unfamiliar experiences
because they are new and challenging and there for
us to explore. We also give up our favoured and
ought-for securities because as we grow, they no
onger satisfy us or because we are pushed or
motivated' to enter new fields, embark on new

discoveries and new ventures of growth an
experience, contact and learning. Once there v
are unable to return to our previously favoure
position – we must go on and not back. This is li
as we know and experience it and only in sleep c
we regress and recapture former territories in ou
dreams.

At such times of growth and exploration, losse
are inevitable, giving an unpleasant reality,
trauma at a different level and challenging ou
sense of invulnerability. A grandparent, siblin,
parent or close friend dies; or a loved pet dies or
killed. With each loss there is grief and a degree c
questioning self-reproach and guilt. Did we lov
them enough? Do enough for them? Treat ther
with the love and sensitivity they deserved? At th
same time our own immortality is put into ques
tion, creating added anguish in the mourning an
loss situation.

Mourning is the reaction to loss and part c
normal grief response to irretrievable loss. Afte
responses of shock, anger, disbelief, self-reproacl
there is depression, insomnia, loneliness, sadnes
and fear. To some extent such feelings come to th
surface again whenever there is the anniversary c
a death, with a varying degree of flatness, sadnes
and sense of vulnerability throughout life.

In a severe case, there may be very severe depre
ssion with absolute insomnia, anorexia and suicida
intent. The person just fails to rally and recovei
whatever treatment is given, and death may follo\
from self-inflicted causes or a fading away and lacl
of reaction in any of the vital organs.

Reaction to another type of loss following an
radical operation, particularly hysterectomy o
mastectomy, may involve a sense of mutilation an

unbearable anguish for some which requires both before such an operation and for a period of at least several months afterwards a very special sensitivity from doctor and family.

A patient with a phobic condition after an acute grief experience described her symptoms to me as never wanting to lose anyone again. She felt quite all right in the company of children. They posed no threat of loss, as she would 'go' first. Her constant nausea was a barrier to closeness and a defence, keeping all others at a 'safe' distance, rejecting, pushing away, to avoid the pain of another loss.

Homoeopathic Answers to Grief

Experienced users of homoeopathy will find helpful Dr Trevor Smith's guide to remedies effective in coping with grief and loss. Use 30c potency. Anyone new to homoeopathy or inexperienced, who is suffering from the symptoms described, should consult a homoeopath who will prescribe the most appropriate remedy and potency.

Aurum met. – Where there is severe, unrousable depression and suicidal intent or the threat of it.

Arnica – For the stage of acute shock, grief and vulnerability, bruised psychologically, weak and unable to cope. Exhaustion. Insomnia.

Baptisia – Where indifference and exhaustion are marked.

Ignatia – One of the best remedies but where there are changeable, hysterical tendencies with tears, sighing and withdrawal and failure to share feelings openly.

Naja – A remedy for the more profound melancholic reaction with hopelessness, defeat and the risk of suicidal impulses.

Natrum mur. – One of the best remedies for tearfu
exhaustion and despair without the dangerous
melancholia of *Naja* and *Aurum*. Usually better
for being left alone but on this occasion wants
someone to be with them in the house.

Natrum sulph. – For mourning where withdrawal
and solitude are marked. Worse in the morning
(*Lachesis*, *Sulphur*). Concentration is lacking and
silent moroseness typical.

Phosphoric acid – The great remedy for mourning
problems with the most profound exhaustion and
fatigue to the extent of prostration and inability to
rally. Tired in bed even when they have slept.

Sepia – Irritable depression with indifference, but
better for people around them. Very negative,
sensitive and usually constipated.

Arsenicum – For the more restless, chilly, agitated,
almost deluded mourning states. Fussy, unable to
rest, worse after midnight.

Lycopodium – For milder forms, with gastric problems, insecurity, anticipating the worst.

28

Tension

One of the commonest emotional problems seen in any surgery is the state of tension, often inseparable from an anxiety state. It is, however, always a physical state with an underlying emotional cause. Commonly there is an awareness of an emotional block, an underlying problem that cannot be dealt with or easily discussed for reasons of the personalities concerned, or because of the limitations of the communication permitted in the relationship.

A real or imagined barrier is present, which cannot be overcome and which is the cause of the tension and heightened feelings, provoking an imbalance in normal muscular relaxation and tone with a mixture of emotional and physiological changes. These form the typical picture of the tension state. Everything is held in that wants naturally to burst out – hence the tension, anxiety and discomfort. Because the smooth, unconsciously controlled muscles respond to the state of health and equilibrium of the emotions, they are the main target and receptors for imbalance and heightened tension, translating emotional blockages and frustrations into physical symptoms.

These occur wherever the unconscious has powerful sphere of physical influence and rep resentation by way of smooth muscles – particu larly affected are the stomach, colon, walls o blood vessels, chest and sometimes the joints c limbs or lower back region.

Restlessness, either physical or emotional i common, leading to the general symptom of physi cal exhaustion and fatigue. Because of the state o agitation, the need to move, change position, t find a comfort that seems to exist nowhere, insom nia is always a problem and adds to the genera anxiety and state of exhaustion. Tension does no cease during the night, and often the person wake to find himself grinding his teeth, and with a fixe jaw and body.

Nightmares are a frequent occurrence, ofte with a feeling of being trapped or attacked, with n possibility of escape, to such a degree at times tha sleep itself is feared, in spite of the fatigue. In th sensitive young child, sleep-walking may occur, th child sometimes impossible to wake.

Backache is common, usually in the low lumba region, often intractable, sometimes chronic, an made worse by a variety of treatments that do no sufficiently acknowledge the underlying emotiona causes and allow them to emerge. This low bac pain also interferes with sleep, as does worry abou indigestion and sometimes constipation. The whol of the intestinal system becomes blocked an sluggish like the mental state. In others the bowel react more violently and there are bouts of diar rhoea which may develop into the more sever colitis when the walls of the intestine ulcerate an blood is present in the stools, with the risk o infection or perforation occurring in a severe state.

In such cases the very physical response seems to become a thing in its own right, cut off from the original tension state, and almost replacing it in significance. The other problem that is common is asthma in the sensitive adult or child. Here again the symptoms may develop a life and energy of their own however the underlying tensions evolve and are treated.

A tension state may become intolerable as tension and emotion which cannot be adequately expressed build up. There may be a complete nervous break-down and, instead of a psycho-somatic state developing as outlined above, there is a sudden catharsis of hysterical screaming, violent behaviour and the risk of a suicidal gesture as an expression of the mixed feelings of rage and tension.

Not uncommonly the tension state is complicated further by its treatment. When the tension is severe, almost invariably the allopathic drug treatment is unsatisfactory, provoking problems of dependence, fatigue, heaviness of waking and lethargy. Tension may be even further heightened by the inevitable tranquillizers, which all too often pose an added problem for the patient by provoking similar side-effects of tension and anxiety to those they aim to relieve.

Build-up

Because of the degree of agitation, the feelings of exhaustion and the inability to concentrate, the patient usually needs a period away from work. As so much of the energy is taken up with anxiety about his symptoms and problems and how to resolve them, a self-centred preoccupation may

219

develop, becoming hypochondriacal if not reso ved. The problem with a chronic tension state always that if it is not resolved within a period several weeks by the release and resolution of th underlying emotional state, the physical symptom become much more set in a pattern, and may b impossible to resolve.

A certain degree of tension and awareness normal in everyone, and is part of healthy anticipa tion and attentiveness. Adrenalin is released t stimulate body tone in anticipation of a challeng or possible action. Lack of tone and tension lead t an unhappy state of flabbiness, a sluggish ungainl posture and lack of energy as opposed to mor compact flowing movements. This lack of tone i associated with accident-proneness, clumsines and often hormonal imbalance, and is an indicatio for such homoeopathic remedies of the carbonat family as *Calcarea* or *Kalium carb*.

The absence of tone is no more healthy than a excess of muscular tone, as is characteristic of th typical tension state. Anger is perfectly normal fo all people yet it is a reaction which is often sup pressed and denied because it is feared. In this wa natural assertiveness is often the victim of ou present upbringing, although essential to health For the majority, it is the total absence of aggres sion which is the major problem provoking th build-up of severe tension states.

The internalization and denial of frustration d not stop the constant release of adrenalin, causin a heightening of body tone, an outpouring of bloo sugar, with no possible outlet for the energy Inevitably, this leads to mental and physical il health, such dangerous conditions as diabetes o peptic ulcer, and general malaise and irritability a

220

ll outlets are denied. This excess of body tension
s always produced by unresolved feelings of
conflict, either conscious or unconscious. The net
result is invariably heightened feelings of
apprehension and a tightening of tension in any
part of the body. The chest, abdomen and back
particularly are prone to the development of pain.

The Constitutional Remedy

I give this initially, whenever possible, to free any
underlying rigidity so that subsequent remedies
have more available energy or charge to allow
them to act. The results are usually obvious to the
patient which naturally increases a state of relaxation, confidence and an increased confidentiality
and trust which allows deeper causes to emerge
and to be looked at.

Natrum mur.

I usually give this remedy in high potency early in
the treatment and inevitably it has to be repeated –
sometimes several times as progress is made. It has
the capacity to reduce withdrawal and isolation, to
reduce fear of others (unless based on a delusional
assumption – when other remedies are indicated)
and to facilitate contact with others, including the
physician. In this way it makes for growth and a
lessening of fear and tension. The 200c potency is
essential.

Argentum nit.

Indicated when there are overriding problems of
obsessional fear or phobia which contribute to the
tension state and prolong it through often long-
standing phantasy ideas and distortions of the

world and others, creating an overwhelming threat to normal functioning and severe tension.

Gelsemium

There is a combination of weakness and fear, especially of anything that is about to happen. This creates unbearable and paralysing tension, exhaustion and often attacks of nervous diarrhoea.

29

The Science of Individualization

Homoeopathy, the science of individualization, is very much in the public eye at the moment. There is enormous and growing interest in this form of alternative medicine. When a person has a cold, the homoeopath doesn't just treat the cold. He treats a type of person and a type of cold. It is very common in a family with four or five children for a cold or 'flu to manifest in various ways. One child may have a high temperature, another night sweats, another an acute throat or earache. Each person, for various reasons, tends to react and respond in their own individual way to a cold, 'flu or an infection of the upper respiratory tract – and each person needs an individual remedy.

Samuel Hahnemann, the founder of homoeopathy, was very much aware of this. The mind is key to man, he emphasized, and if you can understand the psychology and mind of the person, you have the key to healing. This was later stressed by Sigmund Freud and the psychologist Grodeck, about 100 years ago. Hahnemann had established homoeopathy firmly as the science of the indi-

vidual – the whole person – mind and body. N
artificial split was made for the convenience o
theory or dogma – the totality always was consi
dered.

The homoeopath is concerned with the whol
picture, not just a hair or skin problem or eczema
gout or rheumatism. His concern is the form th
ailment takes as well as the type of person, an
how that person reacts. This detailed attention t
human relationships is basic to homoeopathy
But it is an approach which isn't only the pro
vince of the homoeopath. Discovering the whol
person is an essential aspect of all healing, what
ever the specialization.

As in most things, there is nothing new under th
sun and this applies equally to homoeopathy
When Hahnemann discovered homoeopathy in th
middle of the 18th century he was, in fact, bringin
to the fore a very ancient healing principle that hac
been known for at least 2,000 years. In some of hi
major works, Hippocrates, the father of medicine
wrote at length about the principle of 'treating
like by like'. Several centuries later the philosophe
and poet, Paracelsus also referred to this prin
ciple which is expressed by the Latin phrase *similic
similibus curentur*.

Hahnemann was a brilliant scholar, chemist
writer and physician. He was also a sensitive man
rigorously opposed to the often violent medica
treatments of his day, particularly purgation and
blood-letting which were in common use. Early in
his career, soon after qualifying, these principles
caused him to give up formal medicine and he
turned to writing, translation and research. It was
then that his experience of malaria in Hungary –
where he had spent two years as a medical student,

came to influence the course of his life. Whilst translating into German an important book of materia medica by Professor William Cullen, a Scottish physician, he became dissatisfied with what he was translating about the treatment of malaria with quinine bark.

He decided to experiment on himself, and as a healthy person, he took cinchona bark which is a quinine. He found that after a few hours he developed all the classic symptoms of the malaria ague or fever: chilliness, drowsiness, flushed face, sweating, intermittent fever and rigors. The symptoms disappeared as soon as he stopped taking the quinine bark. When he resumed, the symptoms appeared again. He thus became the first 'prover' of a homoeopathic remedy.

This simple experiment alerted him to the possibility that the way remedies act – and the way the quinine had acted – was by stimulating a 'like', or similar, reaction to the illness in the patient. And so the cornerstone of homoeopathic medicine was laid.

No Animals

Painstakingly over a period of 25 years Hahnemann built up a system of remedies based on this same method of 'proving', using healthy volunteers including himself, often his own family and other supporters, frequently doctors. No animal experiments were involved. Most of the initial remedies were from plant sources which were known to be poisonous to the human being – that is, having the ability to stimulate a violent reaction in the body. Each remedy was taken as a simple extract from the plant (the mother tincture) and the various symptoms these stimulated in the healthy person were noted and recorded. Eventually they became Hahnemann's homoeopathic materia medica which initially consisted of 60 remedies available for general use with indications for prescribing. And so from that first experiment with cinchona bark developed the whole system of homoeopathic medicines.

Homoeopathy comes from two Greek words – *Homoios* meaning similar or equal and *Pathos* meaning suffering or sickness: thus, similar suffering or sickness. The homoeopathic principle lays down that suffering or pain should be treated by a remedy which will produce similar symptoms when taken by a healthy person, hence the example of malaria being treated by quinine in its homoeopathic form.

A child who eats berries from the poisonous common hedgerow plant Deadly Nightshade will develop a hot, flushed face, a roaring or beating sensation in the face and ears and a very high temperature. The pupils of the eyes may become dilated and there will probably be a pale area around the mouth. Often with Deadly Nightshade (*Belladonna*) poisoning, very intense pains are felt, particularly in the throat and ears. This is the picture of the toxicology of *Belladonna*. How do we prescribe it?

If a homoeopath is asked to treat a child with the symptoms just described, he would use *Belladonna* homoeopathic remedy. If used in the correct potency, it is usually highly effective and the child is better within a few hours. What can cause illness can also cure, providing it is given in the homoeopathic form.

An overdose of aspirin provokes in the unfortunate person a flushed, purple face and a sensation of banging, hammering or whistling noises in the ears. But aspirin – salicylic acid – in its homoeopathic form is what the homoeopath uses very effectively for tinnitus – 'head noises', often associated with progressive deafness and Menières disease. It is the same homoeopathic principle which applies even in using something like aspirin which in its crude form has toxic side effects.

Poisoning from ergot fungus on wheat or the agaricus toadstool gives rise to similar symptoms – spasm of the peripheral arteries and arterials resulting in whitish/bluish extremities, often with pain, inflammation and swelling akin to frostbite and gangrene. The homoeopath uses both poisons homoeopathically for the effective treatment of severe chilblains and a poor peripheral circulation.

Samuel Hahnemann found that when he used the mother tinctures – the simple extracts from the plants – he noticed the side effects and this worried him. To reduce these effects he began to dilute his remedies and found to his amazement that by doing so he was enhancing the power and efficacy of the remedy. The more he diluted the mother tincture, the more effective the response. This process is called potentization because the remedy is said to be made up in potency through a series of dilutions.

Key Factor

He also found that vigorous shaking of the remedy for a number of seconds between each dilution further increased its power and efficacy. This vigorous shaking (called succussion) uniquely vitalizes the remedy at each stage of its dilution and is an

absolutely key factor in homoeopathy and the pre
paration of the remedies.

Another essential aspect of homoeopathic
medicine is that the patient's symptoms are never
suppressed. To the homoeopath these symptoms
are an expression of the patient's vital being and
his response to stress at the deepest levels within
him. Homoeopathic remedies are only used to
stimulate the awareness and healing response to
the underlying stress.

The concept of constitutional types is a frequent
area of confusion and muddle, because it is often
wrongly assumed that the particular individual is
being type-cast – which is not the case at all.

It has been commonplace in homoeopathy for
many years to link together many of the typical
symptoms of the remedy into a profile characteristic of the overall picture – often one of the 'poly-
crests' which have many different sites of action. In
particular, the mental aspects, metabolic characteristics and physiological reactions and sen-
sitivities are grouped together. These form a series
of remedy-profiles called the constitutional types,
which can be an invaluable aid to prescribing.

Such a concept, however, is only an adjunct and
a guide to the characteristics of the proving picture
of the remedy and toxicology studies. They are *not*
a convenient slot or ad hoc profile, used to group
or type-cast the individual person. When taken
together with the unique overall history and
characteristics of the person, they may be helpful
in the consideration of which particular remedy
best fits the particular person at the time they are
seen.

The concept of constitutional types should never
be used in isolation, as this would only lead to

naccurate prescribing and inevitably unsatisfac-
ory responses to treatment.

World Study

The exact mechanism of action of homoeopathy is
still uncertain, and a matter for research and study
in many centres throughout the world.

Of course, homoeopathy does not act as a
panacea, or cure-all, for every type of illness. Certain problems require a conventional approach,
although at such times, homoeopathy can always
play an important supporting role in stimulating
healing and reducing side-effects and complications. For many conditions, in all age groups,
homoeopathy offers a rapid, first-line treatment,
without complications, often where conventional
methods have failed or have no treatment to offer.

Naturally success depends upon careful diagnosis, sound prescribing and the choice of potencies used in treatment. The results are often aston-
ishing because of homoeopathy's unique action
both upon the deepest psychological levels of the
individual – causing a profound sense of well-being
and energy-release – and in the more specific
symptom-relief of the original complaints.

All cure is from within. Medicines themselves do
not cure. Homoeopathic remedies mobilize the
vital reaction of the person to cure, enabling him to
heal himself. This vital reaction towards cure is in
all of us if we can mobilize it. Homoeopathy is
without doubt one of the most rapid and effective
tools we have which can stimulate a curative
response by the body. It is only in recent years that
the inherent power of the remedies has become
recognized and sought after.

229

30

The Homoeopathic Nosodes

The Nosodes and Emotional Illness

The Indications to prescribe are:

1. A past history of the specific disease.
2. Family history of the specific disease.
3. The mental condition of the patient.

TUBERCULINUM BOVUM
SYPHILINUM
MEDORRHINUM
THE BOWEL NOSODES – Gaertner
                            – Morgan
                            – Sycotico
                            – Dys Co.

CARCINOSIN
PSORINUM
PYROGEN
HYDROPHOBIUM

Nosodes are prepared from pathological material, made up into homoeopathic potency by a series of succussed dilutions for safety and purity and greaer effectiveness of the remedy. The major homoeopathic nosodes are discussed in the following chapter, with especial emphasis on their action on the mentals and their indication in psychological conditions.

Nosodes play a valuable role in the treatment of all chronic illness or any conditions which dates from the specific disease. A patient who has never been well since an attack of Glandular Fever, is likely to require the specific nosode at some time in their treatment. Where there has been a long period of dis-ease, perhaps twenty, even thirty years since a tubercular glandular condition was diagnosed in childhood, or adolescence, it is likely that the specific *Tub. Bov.* nosode will be needed. In general a nosode is only given once in the single dose and this is not repeated for a period of at least six months.

Tuberculinum

Anxious, depressed, defeated, there is a sense of failure. All symptoms are worse in the evening until midnight (*Sepia*). Talkative, the mind is alert and over-active or tormented, especially at night (*Lyc.*). There is an obstinacy about the personality, especially useful for the obstinate child. There is a characteristic desire for change, travel and movement (*Calcarea*, *Calc. phos.*). The mental state is at times bizarre and borders on the schizoid. Symptoms tend to relapse, often associated with a raised temperature in the evenings of an intermittent type. Not uncommonly, there is a strong history of TB in the family, with a dry tickling irritating cough, although all investigations have been consistently negative over the years. They have blue schlerotics typically and often a tuft of hair over the lower spinal lumbar region. Dissatisfied with everything, they are easily described as cosmopolitan because of their rootless feelings. There is reluctance to take on any form of intellectual concentration work, which worsens all symptoms. Suicidal at times, but especially at night when thoughts crowd-in and usually of a depressive nature.

Syphilinum (from primary syphilitic material)

First proved by Swann in 1880.

There is loss of memory, the thoughts confused, can't find the right word, especially for names and recent events (*Medorrhinum*, *Lycopodium*). There is a sense of becoming insane, of everything stopping and being paralysed. They feel removed from everything, indifferent to the future (*Nat. mur.*). Apathy is marked alternating with indifference and worse for consolation (*Nat. mur.*). Fears of the dark (*Medorrhinum*), of being contaminated (*Calcarea*) with marked obsessional features, are a differentiating feature from *Medorrhinum*. There is fear of disease which accounts for the obsessional hand-washing and double-checking. Obsessional doubting is marked. Fear of giving away, of loss of consciousness, of losing control, of anaesthetics. Others know they are unclean. All symptoms are worse at night in contrast to *Medorrhinum*, from sunset to sunrise. Note the marked changes of mood from laughing to weeping without cause (cp. *Ignatia*, *Pulsatilla*). Severe mental retardation. Fear of madness (*Calcarea*, *Cannabis indica*, *Pulsatilla*). Severe melancholia (*Aurum met.*, *Sepia*). Suicidal. Indifferent to friends and there is an absence of joy (*Sepia*). Compulsive, lack of straightforwardness, a compulsive liar and devious to the point of being difficult to prove as such.

Medorrhinum (the gonorrhoeal nosode made from historical material)

The mental state is one of confusion and forgetfulness. Time passes so slowly that they are always in a hurry (*Nux. vom.*). Memory is impaired for dates, facts and events, especially of recent events. There is an impaired ability to concentrate. There are delusional beliefs, often of an anxious paranoid type, especially the belief that someone is just behind them or that others are talking about them. They may have visual hallucinations (*Phosphorus*), everything seems unreal (*Alum*). Weeps when talking and characteristically very changeable (*Pulsatilla*). There is a presentiment of death (*Aconitum*). Fear of the dark and of falling (*Cannabis indica*, *Stramonium*). Fear of poverty. Homesick (*Kali carb.*). As with *Psorinum* and *Sulphur* there is canine hunger with hunger still present after eating. They are also sensitive to reprimand (*Carcinosin*). Suicidal at times (*Aurum met.*). All symptoms are worse in the daytime and for thunder, or better at sunset and at night, and also for being at the seaside, for wet weather and lying on the abdomen.

The Bowel Nosodes

Non-lactose fermenting bacteria, present in the stool in addition to the normal *B. coli* inhabitants proliferate as a result of a vital reaction to dis-ease, rather than causing symptoms. Most of the work was done by Bach, Paterson and Wheeler.

Morgan (Bach)

The key-note is *intensity* with a weepy, irritable, state of mind and fits of temper especially if contradicted (*Nux*). Fear of crowds and hypochondriacal (*Lyc.*). Impulses to suicide by leaping from a high window (*Sulph.*). Fear of death or impending disaster. Congestion is a keynote with congestive headaches. Introspective, he or she avoids company but is worse if alone in the house (*Lyc.*). Note the resemblance to *Lycopodium* in many features.

Gaertner (Bach)

Here the key-note is malnutrition. There is an irritable, quick-tempered condition with hypersensitivity marked, an overactive mind with an undernourished body. Tense, nervous, impatient, jealous or depressed (*Lachesis*). There is a claustrophobic fear of crowds and company.

Dys Co (Bach)

The key-note here is anticipatory anxiety and nervous tension (*Lyc.*). There is a hypersensitivity to criticism and strangers with marked shyness. Physical restlessness and fidgety behaviour is described (*Zinvum met.*).

Sycotico (Paterson)

The key-note is spasm with irritability. Note especially the intense nervous irritability, shyness, fear of the dark, of animals, especially dogs (*Belladonna*). Fear of being alone (*Kali carb.*), twitching, 'live flesh' around the eyes. Bladder irritability with nervous frequency is common.

234

Carcinosin (prepared from cancerous tissue of breast adenoma, Foubister)

One of the most fastidious of all remedies, nervous, determined, intolerant and very competitive. Won't commit themselves with attitudes of sitting on the fence. Obstinacy (cp. *Tub. bov.*). There is prolonged fear, unhappiness and anticipation (*Lycopodium*), sensitive to music (*Aurum met.*, *Tarentula*, *Hisp.*). Better for dancing (*Sepia*). Note the blue schlerotics (*Tub. bov.*).

There is a typical dullness, with thinking difficult or disinterested and an aversion to conversation. *Carcinosin* is linked to *Medorrhinum* for the treatment of backward or mentally defective children. Foubister found it especially indicated for a background of prolonged fear or unhappiness. Fear is present generally with anticipation (*Aconitum*, *Lycopodium*).

There is love of travel (*Tub. bov.*) and better for the sea (*Medorrhinum*). Enjoys thunder (*Sepia*). Sympathy towards others (*Phos.*). Sensitive to reprimand (*Medorrhinum*). Sleeps in the knee-elbow position (*Medorrhinum*, *Calc. phos.*, *Phos.*, *Sepia*, *Lycopodium*).

Psorinum (nosode of the scabies vesicle)

The first nosode, prepared by Hahnemann from scabies vesicle matter and once thought to be a cure for chronic Psora conditions. This was not to be so, but the remedy is of value for the following mental states.

There is an itchy, chilled, neglected, dirty-looking state of despair, constantly sad and depressed. Appetite is excessive canine but they rarely put on weight. Suicidal, religiose, there are strong obsessional features with fixed ideas especially of defeat or failure, bordering on the psychotic or delusional. They nearly always want to be alone. Irritability is marked and like *Sulphur* they are worse for water and washing and even more neglected and unkempt.

Hydrophobium (lyssined saliva of the rabid dog)

The key-note here is hypersensitivity to an extreme degree. All symptoms are aggravated by dazzling lights, the sight, sound or even the thought of fluid or running water. Increased libido to an uncontrollable and painful degree. The typical tension headaches are worse for emotion or bad news.

Pyrogen (putrefying raw beer, originally by Drysdale)

Restlessness is marked with constant agitation. Always on the move despite marked prostration and exhaustion. Overtalkative, with mental confusion and disturbance of body-image. The whole body seems to spread out and cover the bed. Feels divided, as if two people. The bed feels too hard (cp. *Arnica*, *Baptisia*). Delusions of wealth and grandeur. A sense of general numbness in the whole body, spreading everywhere. Note the racing of mind, thinking and talking faster and faster. Irritable delirium, with the eyes closed – sees a man at the foot of the bed. With the head on the pillow, does not know where the rest of the body is. Buoyancy of spirits, muttering delirium, general horror, insomnia.

31

Schizophrenia

Speaking for a moment as a beekeeper; at a time of year when the nectar-flow is at the full, my homing flight towards the hive of schizophrenia, with all its patterns of organization and disorganization, will be via several already well-foraged gardens. However, the pollen there is somewhat tempting, and I shall pause to hover over so-called 'normal' social interaction; exploring briefly in passing, the 'stamens' of neurosis and its therapy, before delving into those layers and vicissitudes which emerge as the psychotic mind.

Beginning with the corner stone of homoeopathic medicine, namely the principle of the similimum, which has been referred to since the time of Hippocrates and later by Paracelsus, Hahnemann developed this ancient concept into a scientific body of clinical knowledge, based on sound working principles which could be used in a clinical situation, both to treat the patient, and to predict the outcome of treatment with precision.

All great truths and basic principles of man are true, not only in the particular situation, but also in other more general aspects of man's being. That is to say it is likely that the similimum principle in homoeopathy is but one aspect of a general simillimum principle, which expresses itself not only in our choice of remedy and approach to the patient, but also in other broader areas of man's expression. Here I want to concentrate in particular on its relevance to the workings of the mind, and to lead on to thinking about its meaning and relationship to the schizophrenic process.

By way of approach, therefore, I want to develop the hypothesis, based on clinical experience and observation, that the simillimum principle is clearly to be seen at various levels of expression of man's psychological health and maturity. The concepts I have in mind will, I hope, become immediately clear to you when I remind you of what I call –

(1) *The social or 'normal' simillimum principle*

This is both the expression of unresolved emotional material in ordinary social situations, and attempts to come to terms with it. The analyst calls it 'working through' in a social situation. We are concerned with the formation of, for example, siblings; parental figures; allies; figures of rivalry; love, or jealousy, in such day-to-day happenings as are familiar to everyone. Office tensions between 'personalities', the difficulty of doing any work in certain group situations, such as the committee, or board room, where emotional material so frequently comes to the fore, at the expense of work and the task at hand, creating frustration and involving an excessive amount of time for what would otherwise be a simple matter. W. R. Bion referred extensively to this problem in his works on group inter-action and group dynamics. The individual creates in such a setting, replicas of the figures and tensions of earlier significant events, perhaps traumatic at the time, or emotionally overwhelming and damaging. The similimum concept is that once this has been re-created in the social situation, unless excessive and over-intense, the individual has a possibility of growth and coming-to-terms with hitherto unresolved parts of himself, without creating a neurosis, or symptoms which would limit or handicap him, or his relationships.

(2) *The social or 'neurotic' similimum principle*

This is the expression of the neurosis, differing only from the social similimum by the intensity and excess of feelings which are expressed in both work and social situations. Because of this excess, normal growth and 'working-through' is no longer possible, and there is a tendency to group-alienation. All the ingredients of the earlier trauma are re-created around the self to produce the neurotic similimum, but because of the neurosis-tendency to compulsive repetition and excess reaction, growth and maturation are at best very slow, as compared with the more benign social similimum situation.

(3) *The therapeutic similimum principle*

This is a contrived treatment situation, using the environment, the terms of reference of the treatment situation, and the presence of the therapist, to artificially re-create the earlier neurotic similimum more effectively than in the social situation.

239

Because of the therapist's intervention the neurosis emerges more clearly and is acceptable, as opposed to any meaningful or useful emergence within the social situation. Growth can, therefore, take place and symptoms are relieved. I am thinking here of such treatment-situations as abreaction in the treatment of shell-shocked troops, and rehabilitation techniques. Also hypnosis, drama and group therapy, and finally in individual analytic treatment, when the relationship with the therapist re-creates the similimum in the transference situation.

(4) *The psychotic similimum principle*

This is a non-event because of the severity and intensity of the illness and the fragmented world of the schizophrenic. The ego, or in simpler terms, the self of the individual, is unable to re-create earlier trauma in any sort of a whole or meaningful way. That is to say, neither in the social nor the neurotic-therapeutic way. Everything is fragmented within, and these fragments of self, mind and phantasy, are then projected outwards, and experienced as being totally outside the self, and alien to it. Thus is created a threatening, bewildering, kaleidoscopic world of fact, phantasy, delusion, hallucination, suspicion, with the frequent occurrence of ideas of reference. The integrative knitting-together harmoniously of earlier trauma cannot occur, because the whole drive of the schizophrenic is towards the outside, with resulting splitting, fragmentation, disharmony and chaos of both self and self-images and boundaries.

The late Morris Robb, in a paper on psychosis and homoeopathy, also referred to integrity, which he defined as wholeness and that 'completeness of the psychic self'.

The core of schizophrenia is damage to the ego feeling, or ability to differentiate self from environment. This is the prime area of damage, the patient experiences inner and external sensations as a continuum, and no barrier between them.

The psychotic cannot effect a similimum cure in the psychological situation because he denies its very existence, by pulverizing both the experiences of the outer world, together with the inner elements of the mind, into fragments; and these fragments include the self; identity, knowing who one is and who is other. The essential nature of schizophrenia is this external projection of self and reality into outside situations, creating a break with reality, and a world of delusion. This is to be compared with depression, often associated with a feeling of being dead inside and generally emotionally flat and empty. Here there is destruction, and possibly fragmentation of the self and the images within the mind, but there is no severe projection and therefore no break with reality, unless the depression becomes psychotic in type and intensity. It is, therefore, this basic splitting and projection which is responsible for all the bizarreness of the schizophrenic, his inappropriateness, hallucinations, and feeling on a different wavelength. His external world is not re-creating sibling rivalry; parental figures in the work-group; but rather those fragments of self and similimum-matrix are perceived in the environment, and inside others, who are felt to contain recognizable bits of himself within their living envelopes. Only when these fragments of self can be recognized and acknowledged as part of the ego, by the reverse of projection, that is to say, the process of internalization, can a cure be effected, and the psychic self become intact again with a possibility of normal similimum 'working-through' to occur in a therapeutic situation, and eventually a social one.

Robb stated that schizophrenia was dependent upon internal or external object relationships, and that these were absent in deepest sleep, which is characterized particularly by an absence of dreaming. In this situation there can be no fragmentation or distortion because there are no objects. He emphasized the important fact that this area of deep sleep, with its void of object relationships, is an important part of man's twenty-four hour daily cycle. He puts forward the interesting hypothesis that the modus operandi and therapeutic potential of certain physical treatments, which were previously 'fashionable', such as ECT, or insulin therapy, was to induce what he called a 'stunned sleep', or 'toxic sleep', which resembles this object-free sleep, where there can be no transposition or fragmentation of objects.

Robb again sees the essential nature of the psychotic experience, as investing inner phantasy objects and thoughts and imaginations with an external concrete reality, whilst he invests reality and external object material with a dream-like quality; he thus confuses these external and internal worlds.

One of the problems of the psychotic, is that anyone in contact with the schizophrenic becomes, to some extent, part of his delusional system and phantasy world, where there is frequently suspicion and mistrust. The homoeopath treating the patient has, therefore, the difficult problem of overcoming this barrier, to enable him to contact more amenable parts of the self, which can respond to the therapeutic approach.

I would like now to consider my general homoeopathic approach, having taken into account the failure or non-existence of the ubiquitous similimum principle in the schizophrenic.

I start from the belief that in all life and all creatures there is both life and death represented; both light and shade; negative and positive. That all of us contain a tendency to being both self-destructive, as well as creative, in our urges and expressions.

In the psychotic patient, no matter how disturbed, there are periods when he is sensible, when he is able to, or chooses to, make contact, both appropriately and in a meaningful way with his environment. During that time he exists as an entity and as a person, recognizing me as an entity and as a person, who is separate from him. He senses his existence. It is true that this sense of totality-of-existence, of being a person in his own right, is weak, maybe transitory, and fragmentary, but it is nevertheless a well-recognized fact. This is the basis of my first and most important approach which is namely to recognize, acknowledge, and strengthen the positive integrating part of the self without denying the sick side. I attempt to build a bridge of trust and openness between myself and the unfragmented ego, in order that we can discuss and relate anything he and I consider relevant. I personally find it very useful to discuss both dream and hallucinatory material, as these both interest and concern him, and often create anxiety and confusion. Whatever is related I accept, and attempt to discuss in terms of the fragmentation process; at the same time always laying emphasis on the healthy move towards integration and cure even though this may not be obvious during an acute phase of flare-up. Often the dreams give a clue to how the integrative side of the patient is coping with the onslaught of fragmentation and madness.

Freeman, when he talks of the ego disturbances of the chronic schizophrenic, says that this is not just a mysterious process of the disease, having no correspondence with normal experience, labelling the psychotic as a creature of another bizarre world, alien to our own. On the contrary, these are phenomena experienced in many normal situations outside psychosis, and particularly when the capacity for self-perception is lessened. There is a continuum from clear-cut ego-awareness, to merging into the external environment, and fluctuations of ego-feeling in a variety of states, in us all.

My second and combined approach is to prescribe homoeopathically, and according to the classical Hahnemennian similimum principle. The patient is always examined physically and a careful history is taken from both the patient and his family.

Before proceeding to more definite, clear-cut homoeopathic prescribing, I would like to give you three examples of hallucinatory material from a twenty-three-year-old schizophrenic girl, with a four-year history of agoraphobia, fear of women – especially her mother, hearing voices for six months, and feeling that people were talking about her. During treatment sessions she was largely silent much of the time, often smiling and giggling inappropriately, looking upwards, and listening. On questioning, at the fourth meeting, the content ɔf the auditory hallucinations was as follows – Let's get together'; 'The doctors stink'; and finally Eat, don't talk, eat!'.

My brief comments about 'Let's get together' were, that these were representative of an integrating, getting-together, that is to say, a healing and healthy part of the self which was trying to repair the split in the mind and to overcome the confusion in order to bring her back together as one entity – to make sense of her illness, and to facilitate healing. I said that because of the pain of her illness, she put and experienced parts of herself outside her, and these were experienced as voices, which wanted to come back inside, so that she could become a whole and complete person again. The more direct transference interpretation of her getting together with me was ignored, as I considered it most important to acknowledge those impulses to heal or undo the split within herself at this time.

The second piece of hallucinatory material, namely 'The doctors stink', was interpreted as her ill-self, which she experienced as being bad and rotten and unloving, i.e. 'stinking', and it was this which she was projecting into the doctors; including myself, pushing them away, making them undesirable. By making me 'stink', she was denying this unloved part of herself, and at the same time attempting to undo the good feelings referred to above, and thereby to negate the getting-together.

The third hallucination, 'Eat, don't talk, eat!' was designed to make herself a receptacle for food – a sort of dust-bin non-person, an envelope for food, rather than for thoughts, needs, impulses and feelings. She was very obese, having an unhealthy, greasy skin, and this worried her. She would like to

245

have been slim like her younger sister, who was a full-time student. Talking and words were ways of making contact with people and the outside world, but she distrusted people, including myself at present. By eating at the expense of talking she was running away from expressing herself more clearly, which could lead us into greater understanding, coming-together, and eventual cure.

Homoeopathy is always helpful in schizophrenia, in certain cases it is curative. Most of the cases I have treated have shown a lessening of the over-activity. Frequently the sleep disturbances have improved markedly. It is not uncommon to see a rapid lessening of the hallucinations, as the patient begins to take an interest in her self-appearance, frequently neglected in the acute phase of the illness. Often they are worried, particularly if they are young and adolescent, about their skin, hair, weight and general appearance. It is common to see an improvement in the health of the skin and hair at an early stage, with a lessening of acne. This is reassuring for the patient, as they feel they have the possibility of improvement, and that their bodies are not 'rotten and stinking'. There may be a disturbance of body-image, as in anorexia nervosa – often a border-line schizophrenic problem, and all too frequently part of a subtle delusional system.

I am going to initially consider adolescent schizophrenia. The skin is often damp, and the extremities icy cold. Frequently there is a greasy quality to the skin, particularly that of the forehead, chin, shoulders and back, where acne may be severe. Dandruff is common, and a cause of anxiety in the adolescent, who is still gaining confidence in their external image. Obesity is frequent in one form of adolescent schizophrenia, usually with an associated liking for greasy fatty foods, and it is particularly this type of patient, referred to above, who may use their bodies as dust-bins, being totally undiscriminating in what they eat – this as compared with the fastidiousness of the anorexic.

In a rather bulky, flabby, greasy-skinned girl with icy cold extremities and a damp sweaty skin, it is important to remember *Calcarea*, particularly if there is a combination of constant fidgety over-activity, associated body weakness, and pallor. These patients are usually thirsty, and drink tea or coffee, often heavily sweetened, throughout the day, and are always to be found hugging the radiators. *Calc. Sulph.* may be indicated where the patient is warmer, very untidy, and has an early morning aggravation. This is a useful remedy when there is the paleness and bulk of *Calcarea*, together with the sweaty heat and fat-craving, which is so characteristic of *Sulphur*.

Very slim anorexic girls, wasting away because of obsessional food-phobias, and a grossly distorted body-image, with very cold and damp, frequently blue, hands and feet and symptoms of weakness and fatigue, when there is an associated problem of chronic infection in the sinuses or throat – often respond to *Silicea*, which is the chronic of *Pulsatilla*.

When the menstrual cycle is weak and irregular, and the flow scanty and short-lived, in a compliant non-aggressive girl with a tendency to weep, better for sympathy, and when the symptoms and mood vary from day to day – *Pulsatilla* is usually the remedy of choice. Frequently these patients are quite intolerant of fats, and thirstless, as compared

247

to the *Calcarea* patient, who sips throughout the day, or may chew such bizarre things as chalk or soap. In the treatment of schizophrenia, whatever remedy is given, it must always be based on two considerations – this has priority over all other factors and must determine the treatment and choice of the homoeopathic similimum. Of primary importance is to choose that remedy which best fits the presenting dominant mental symptoms at the time of the prescription, and also the main physical characteristics, symptoms and modalities which are unique for that patient when seen. The constitutional remedy for the patient is the second most important consideration. This may or may not be the same remedy as outlined above. It is, however, always of immense value and should be prescribed for the patient at an early date in the treatment. The actual discerning of this remedy may be veiled by the psychotic process, and its choice may only be manifest when there has been an improvement in the acute picture, particularly when the patient is hyper-manic. The family may provide an important clue as to the choice of constitutional remedy when the patient is unable to be of help, or is unco-operative. In my experience the homoeopathic remedy pushes the patient forward sufficiently to allow the therapist to relate more easily to the healthy parts of the ego. The patient responds, not only at a mental, but also at a physical level, thus fostering the relationship between the doctor and healthy personality fragments.

Paschero, in a 1975 paper on mental symptoms in homoeopathy, states that the homoeopathic similimum stimulates the natural forces of fundamental man, making possible the rectification of his vital senses, and the similimum is directed to a more perfect emotional adaptation to the human world. Both Robb and Paschero emphasize empathy and its importance. Paschero is most stimulating when he states that the constitutional homoeopathic remedy, when correctly applied, may be the solution to the biological problem which Freud so urgently demanded in the course of some of his more difficult psycho-analytic cases.

This is a further example of case material: for simplicity, from a non-schizophrenic person:

The patient, aged 30, came with two acute haemorroids, purple, inflamed, the size of small plums. She had been unable to sit down for about a week, also had been tearful and depressed for several months. She was given her constitutional remedy, which was *Pulsatilla*. After several hours the patient suddenly felt more confident, able to express herself more freely and clearly, and could talk-out old resentments and repressed angers. Almost immediately the depression cleared and did not recur. The haemorroids had also totally cleared-up after one week, and were no longer visible on examination. I take this as an example of how the homoeopathic similimum is able to mobilize blocked and repressed parts of the ego-responses, and to create a very rapid cure, confirming Paschero's concepts, referred to above.

In considering basic remedies of value in the treatment of psychosis, Nash describes the triad of *Belladonna*, *Hyoscyamus* and *Stramonium* to be helpful particularly in the over-active manic cases, differing rather in degree of excitability than in other more detailed aspects of the psychosis. *Belladonna* is made from the entire Deadly Nightshade plant at the time of flowering in Summer. I

249

have not found it to be of particular use, unless
there is a pseudo-psychosis secondary to infection
or alcoholism. There is always a remittent fever
and the particular characteristics are redness of the
skin, in particular of the face; heat and dryness
and a feeling of burning. The pulse is bounding and
it is a remedy most indicated when there is violent
maniacal excitement, with great restlessness, delusions and hallucinations. In that situation it is
well-indicated and a good response may be
expected.

Stramonium, made from the entire plant of the
Thorn Apple, covers many of the most problematic
symptoms of schizophrenia. It is of value when
there are violent bouts of excitability, extreme
restlessness, and agitated delusional activity. In
differentiating it from *Belladonna*, there is usually
a continuous fever in the patient, as opposed to the
remittent type of *Belladonna*, and the patient is
also very talkative, and over-active to an extreme
degree.

Hyoscyamus – the extract of the whole plant of
Henbane – has mania with no fever, and its great
characteristic is a passive delirium with hallucinations, suspicion and obsessional features. The
patient lies picking at the bedclothes, usually
totally inaccessible to reality.

Tarantula Hispania – again the extract of the
entire insect, found along the Mediterranean coast.
It is the most destructive of all schizophrenic
remedies, useful where there is a combination of
soiling, tearing of sheets or clothes, damage to
furniture, and attempts to destroy the self in a
highly dangerous way. There is excessive change of
mood, often quite rapidly, with swings from

ypermania to the depths of despair. They are always very agitated.

Psora is that inherited, miasm or ghost of illness running through families, which Hahnemann described in his work on chronic disease. Psora has many bizarre chronic refractory symptoms, especially it has mental disease and delusions of all kinds. In refractory non-responsive disease, it must never be forgotten, and of all the anti-Psora remedies, probably *Sulphur*, and *Psorinum* – the nosode, are of enormous value. *Causticum* has also proved to be of value, but I would recommend in particular the first two remedies, particularly in those cases when well-indicated remedies fail to stimulate a response.

Thuja Occidentalis, the tree of life, is prepared from the young leaves picked at the end of June. This is a well-tried remedy which has many bizarre and hypochondriacal symptoms. Depression predominates and they tend to be agitated, anxious, often irritable people, with fixed delusional ideas. They feel that their body is brittle, transparent and is made of glass and that it will break with the least shock. Or they may feel that they have a living animal in their bowels. Other odd and bizarre sensations are of pain in small localized spots 'like a nail being driven through the head'. They feel they are being influenced by a superior power. The association of Fig-Warts or Condylometa or recent vaccination confirms the remedy.

Anacardium Orientale – made from the fruit of the tree – has hallucinations, and a feeling of split personality, feeling divided by contradictory impulses. He feels controlled, commanded by an external force. There are many strange obsessional features, and loss of memory is very common. The patient laughs inappropriately at hallucinatory voices. There are two strange and peculiar symptoms which are diagnostic: (1) a feeling of having a plug in the inner parts – either head, chest, navel or anus; (2) a feeling that he has a hoop around his body.

Suspicion, paranoia, combined with mild over-activity and an inability to tolerate pressure about the neck or chest makes one consider *Lachesis* This remedy is prepared from the snake venom of the South American Bushmaster. It is characteristic that the patient sleeps into an aggravation and the symptoms and hallucinations are always worse in the morning. They are melancholic, very talkative people with many delusional ideas. Often, associated left-sided body symptoms are also present.

Argentum Nitrum – is a valuable remedy when phobic anxiety symptoms dominate the picture. It is the best remedy for a terrified, over-anxious patient, who is very fearful of the hallucinations, and may be severely claustrophobic or agoraphobic. This remedy may often be needed at a later stage of treatment before confidence is fully established and when social rehabilitation is being planned.

Sepia – prepared from the inky juice of the Cuttle Fish – I have found to be of value, particularly in those patients dragged down by their symptoms, angry and indifferent to their family and loved ones, often resentful and refusing to allow them to visit. There is an absence of joy. The psychosis is frequently puerperal in origin. They are usually unable to cry and their skin is sallow

nd mottled, with constipation and dragging-down
uterine symptoms, such as a prolapse.

Usually there are no clear-cut causative factors,
but occasionally there has been an acute traumatic
origin leading to a paranoid illness, e.g. loss of an
arm or limb in an industrial accident. I once treated
a steeple-jack, who had his arm amputated after a
crush injury, leading to an acute and severe paranoid illness. *Arnica* and *Allium Cepa* were both
helpful in the management of this case. Often the
onset is insidious however, and each case must be
treated according to its merits and specific
symptom-picture.

Certainly they are not easy to manage, and a
period of institutionalization may be required. A
good relationship with the family, for outside
confirmation of progress in the treatment, and
manifestation, of the delusional process, is helpful.

The results of cases seen have been encouraging,
and often the response has been quite soon after
homoeopathic treatment has been commenced.
The prognosis is usually better when there has not
been a prolonged period of in-patient therapy and
hospitalization, and where electro-shock has not
further changed and complicated the presenting
pattern of the disease.

R. D. Laing, in his moving and thought-
provoking book – 'The Politics of Experience',
describes the schizophrenic process as essentially a
journey into the self through uncharted seas of the
deepest and most dangerous areas of the Id and the
unconscious Ego. He describes clinical material
from patients in analytic therapy, and how they
emerge with greater depths of knowledge and
insight into themselves, as people and into their

253

own motivations. In order to voyage through such uncharted waters, there must be a ship, a primitive rudder or compass of some sort, to escape sinking into total chaos, however simple – however much a Kon Tiki raft. It is this directional element, provided by the therapeutic approach of patient nonjudgemental empathy, together with the similimum remedy, that gives sails and shape to the embryonic remnants of the self, to emerge as the nucleus of a healthier, more balanced and aware self.

I begun with the metaphor of the bee-hive and perhaps you will allow me to end with it. The success of the harvest of the apiary depends not only upon the climate and season, but also upon such attentions as winter feeding when food reserves are low, and providing sufficient summer space and wax, for growth to occur, avoiding the loss of the swarm whenever possible.

So also with the schizophrenic, the patient needs nurturing, support and feeding, by the emphatic holistic approach of the physician, supported by the homoeopathic prescription. He needs room for growth and exploration of self, both his inner and outer worlds, in particular as improvement occurs.

References

Bion, W. R. *Experience in Groups*. Tavistock Publications, 1961.

Freeman, T., Cameron, J. L., McGhie, A. *Chronic Schizophrenia*. Tavistock Publications, 1958.

Laing, R. D. *Politics of Experience*. Penguin Books, 1967.

Nash, E. B. *Leaders in Homeopathic Therapeutics*. Third Indian Edition, 1962.

Paschero, Thomas. *Mental Symptoms in Homeopathy*. Jubille Congress L.M.H.I., 1975.

Robb, Morris. 'The Psychotherapy of Psychotics'. *British Homoeopathic Journal* (April, 1965).

32

The Gentle Kitten

The reasons for writing any book are many and complex, and not just for the personal satisfaction involved. This is always present to some degree – but is the most superficial reason and there are more relevant and deeper causes to consider. First and foremost, there is the urgent need to inform the public, including the patient and his or her doctor that homoeopathy exists as something of real relevant value and merit for their consideration – a method to try and to use, in an easy practical even pleasant way and one that is available – not just something to be read about or mulled over. The philosophy, methodology, approach to the patient and the holistic concepts are all important, but secondary to practical considerations and recommendations, as a stimulus to the reader to try out for himself and the family at least some of the basic potencies.

In general I have tried to communicate two major themes – my personal vision of homoeopathy, its depths, ability to work directly on the psychological processes, the enormous potential to stimulate change and balance and to act in harmony with the deepest inspirational-creative

255

aspects of man for greater happiness and health But the reader above all, must be given mor understanding of the approach, particularly to family first-aid situations. The reader like the patien needs to have certain basic information that is no always easily available – how to match th remedies with the symptoms of the patient; th importance of the modalities or modifying factors the profiles of the most common home remedies how they are made up and should be taken; thei action, and how they should be stored. More know ledge is also needed about diet, its role in health and just what to eat or cut-down on when taking the remedies, and finally having chosen the remedy, what potency to use.

One of my preferred definitions of homoeopathy was given by Jerome K. Jerome in a delightful little book – *Idle Thoughts for an Idle Fellow*, where he describes time as the greatest of all homoeopathic prescribers. Time is important – both for the initia as well as the subsequent consultations. It is essen tial that nothing be pressurized so that a full, deep personal and relevant history can be taken with adequate time for the patient to relate and give their story in depth with any known trigger factors or causes in detail, as also the family history. But above all time is needed for cure, so that the well-prescribed remedy can run its course, the potency act as an impetus and a boost to cure, in this way the vitality, inevitably bound-up and lost to the patient, can be freed again.

We have potentized sunlight as *Sol*, useful in the treatment of many conditions where sunlight plays a role or aggravates, as in certain light-sensitive allergic eczemas and skin conditions or in sunstroke or sunburn. *Luna* is potentized moonlight

256

energy, also of value in certain emotional states and for hay-fever, thread-worm and sometimes asthma. A case could be made out for potentizing time – time 6 perhaps for conditions where it passes too slowly – in the early hours from insomnia or depression, where counting sheep seems endless and when other remedies which have this characteristic like *Medorrhinum*, are not indicated. But the pharmacist would have a difficult problem and need to prepare differently for those who experience time as racing and rushing, always in short supply, when there is never enough of it, making one think of remedies which are always in a hurry, like *Lycopodium*, where everything is done clumsily, and at the last minute. Other remedies with this same rubric are *Belladonna*, *Stramonium* and *Hyoscyamus*. But perhaps after all, it is not such a good idea and we should keep time for the consulting room, for the remedy to run its course and to support the patient when an instant cure is not forthcoming.

Homoeopathy is also related to another favourite book of mine, Lewis Carroll's *Through the Looking Glass*, where the remedy, like the naughty black kitten of Alice, tugs and pulls at the ball of constitutional yarn, rolling back unravelling, like a gentle kitten, pulling and tugging without stopping. Homoeopathy unravels biologically, always in tune with the patient's needs and abilities at the time, without imposing artificial stresses or iatrogenic pressures. The ball symbolizes the patterns of individual experiences and characteristics as well as resistance, built-up over the years, the vitality and vicissitudes of health, as well as of illness, so that a constitutional scroll or calendar is established within the yarn, with which the patient's constitutional can work and resonate, to bring back balance and cure.

The wool symbolizes too, the inter-weaving of genetic inheritance and any weak areas, as well as the results of past pressures or illness. But the black kitten can also have sharp claws at times when it clings precariously to our lap, and homoeopathy can have its sharp edges for a time, as many who have had first hand experience of a healing aggravation will know – before an improvement occurs – the crisis anticipating a turn in the internal dynamics, as the prescribed remedy leads on to the benefits of cure. This is often a time when reassurance is particularly important and explanation of the action of the remedies most needed.

Illness can also be seen like a ball of wool, where the ingredients of our lives have become too tightly bound together, intense, rushing and tearing, meeting deadlines, making time for others, but never enough for personal needs, at a cost to essential rest and relaxation, even to food and nourishment. The aim is to be perfect, too good, to do too much, not wanting to say 'no', often with feelings of misplaced guilt or unexpressed anger and ambivalence.

A patient of 26 described this clearly. She had a diagnosed condition on x-ray of two peptic ulcers and a hiatus hernia. She said she was too tense and 'het-up', too irritable – annoyed with everyone and anyone in her way. Most days she had bouts of temper, critical of others around her and 'pulling them over the coals'. She cannot pause, never sits or takes it easy, cleaning and dusting, but nothing must be touched or moved afterwards, once arranged. She is too fussy, always running after people before she can relax, opening the window of the bathroom or cleaning after others, then rushing in again to polish the mirror, or hoovering - before she can sit down. The washing-up must be done immediately after tea and the wellies put away – the big things, she explained, like wall-papering and painting can wait – until tomorrow. Making the bed, cleaning the car, keeping the books of her business up to date, nothing can be delayed or put-off in the slightest way, because she is perfectionist with herself and also in her demands on others. Another patient who had a stress problem, always pushing herself too much, winds down by thinking of a rhyme her daughter taught her – 'Stay loose, Mother Goose'. But for many, this is not possible and a balancing support-ing background influence is absent.

All of this winds up the ball too tightly, creating a knotted-up internal situation which cannot be easily expressed, let alone resolved. At the same time it must be controlled and contained for the sake of 'keeping up the image and appearances'. Here we have all the typical ingredients of a recipe for a minor or major blow-out or disaster, like tripping-up or twisting the ankle, a nasty fall, brak-ing too hard on a wet and slippery road leading to severe bruising, fracture or dislocation. At other times there is a nasty cut or burn in the kitchen from inattention, perhaps a sudden spasm of indi-gestion, or a cold or attack of flu. Such self-inflicted excesses, over the months and years, form a knot-ted kernel to illness and make for chronic recurrent problems at multiple levels.

Homoeopathy works by unravelling and easing just such tension factors within the hard ball of the constitutional self – in the body with sometimes clearly palpable knots and tensions in certain muscle groups or organs, but also unlocking knots within the mind. As the kitten playfully tugs at the wool until it comes to an end, so homoeopathy brings to the surface every previous situation which at the time was over-intensive, out-of-tune or balance with the individual totality. Provided this natural emergence is not interfered with by a hasty change of remedy, the well-chosen potency will slowly and surely undo any knots within the strands of the individual schema that do not need a mechanical or surgical approach. Once unwound, the hardness and tensions lessened, they can then become much more loosely organised and brought together with less compactness and tightness.

Just as homoeopathy rolls back the patterns of past negative inharmonious happenings, experiences, reactions or attitudes, which affected the constitutional balance adversely – many genetically induced, but others provoked by chance and especially by self-inflicted impositions – so these must also re-emerge during the course of treatment. They occur as minor symptoms and mild exacerbations or aggravations, unless at the time they were of insufficient intensity to form symptoms or problem areas of significance. Some of the crosses the homoeopathic patient has to bear are the temporary re-experiencing of the past – often as periods of exhaustion, a sore throat, common cold, back-ache or recurrence of a past problem or pain, reflecting where an extra twist was given to the yarn and adding to already existing pressures.

Illness is often an exit or emergency situation, one where the patient is more ready for cure and to accept treatment, when the right homoeopathic remedy can gain entry and start to work to reverse n unfavourable trend of the past. This gives a real possibility for a more relaxed mature totality, which is the basic essential for health. In this way, he or she can become more in tune with each situation as it occurs, able to respond more easily and for more creative ways of thinking and being. As there is less pressure, there is more time, more space between the strands of each happening, so that every encounter becomes an individual response, making for greater humour, relaxation and health. This is what the constitutional prescription can do, given the right remedy for the patient's totality in the right potency. In general, the greater the tension and hardness of attitudes, the tighter the ball or the constitutional set, the higher the potency needed, and often the longer it must be allowed to run, especially once the right remedy for the patient has been found and prescribed.

In general a remedy should not be interfered with unless there are good reasons to do so, because it will run, pull and tug at the acquired patterns, until it has either run out of vitality or a cure has been reached. If the remedy does run out of steam, but has been working well until then, with real gains and improvement for the patient, then the kitten is only tired and the same remedy needs re-prescribing in the same or higher potency. If however there is still some aspect or remnant of the ball to unravel, the patient now experiencing new or changed symptoms, with different problems to the original ones, then a new remedy is indicated at this point. In Lewis Carroll's terms, it is time for the white kitten to take over from the black one.

None of us can avoid all the strains of modern living, the pressures of others, their demands, as well as the ones we impose upon ourselves. But

261

such pressures can be more lightly woven ar worn. The strands should lie less intensively, mo: like a skein of wool than a tight ball, loose wrapped and wound in everything we are doing in our talking as in our listening. Whatever th situation, we should not be knotted tight balls, b more resilient and in this way, more resistant an less vulnerable. The over-determined position, lik the hard attitude is indicative of a tense, wound-u personality. It is these attitudes which make fc increased susceptibility to disease, illness an accident-proneness, as well as to all the diseases c civilization. Two major homoeopathic remedie come to mind in this respect. One is *Natrum mu:* which has the hard ball physically as a lump or ba in the throat, but shuns or hates other people an seeks to avoid them. The other is *Nux vomica* which is also typically a hard-ball type in many c its attitudes, with outbursts of irritable spasm, bu it needs others, albeit to argue with them, in black mood of short-fuse intensity.

Homoeopathy is not alternative to conventiona methods, although often wrongly thought of in thi way. This approach is often required, valuable an essential, but homoeopathy can be a very effectiv way of dealing with the many day to day, acut family problems for the self-prescribing lay person especially where a homoeopathic doctor is no available or can be contracted by telephone fo advice when a full consultation is not needed.

In this way, homoeopathy has an importan social role to play, by helping to cut down anc reduce, the enormous expenditure of the Nationa Drug Bill, swollen by expensive and also unnecess ary repeats of tranquillizers, sedatives and often antibiotics that are neither needed nor effective. I an also help to ease the demands on the work load of the busy doctor in the general practice surgery, the casualty and emergency departments. But above all homoeopathy is about an individual approach to an individual patient by an individual doctor – that is why homoeopathy has been called the science of individualization.

Homoeopathy is also a treatment which is essentially ecological in action – one which is in tune with the patient's inner biological environment and does not impose strain upon his outer one either. The method does not lead to an accumulation of toxic dangerous chemicals, nor does it form potentially lethal side or by-products, which put the family in jeopardy. A bottle of homoeopathic pills can safely be taken by the most curious or inquisitive over-active child without risk to health. The most way-out teenager is unlikely to get a buzz from homoeopathy, even where *Cannabis Ind.* or *Opium* have been prescribed, because it is the energy of the original substance that is used and not toxic material in substantial dosage. The most depressed of adults, will not find a suicidal exit by taking an overdose of the remedies, as a way out of life's realities, nor do the remedies cause wasteful addiction or dependency problems. A confused senile elder of the family will not be harmed by mistaking the remedies for his bottle of aperients or sweets. In this way homoeopathy is an ecological therapy, as well as a biological and individual one.

It is important that every book for the general public should stress the safety, ease of use and value of homoeopathy for the family as a whole. But not just books are needed however, also help and support from the local societies, to give talks and create a forum for questions, explanation and discussion – to inform all who are unaware of the existence of the homoeopathic approach to illness and its prevention. We need to stimulate more public awareness by education, using simple straightforward ways, giving positive examples of the method, perhaps from the patients themselves. It is not expensive to purchase the remedies, which are readily available. There is an urgent need to inform that homoeopathy is not a second class treatment but a well-tried approach to illness.